AF361529

ATOMIC COLLECTIVE

Radioactive Life in Kazakhstan

In the aftermath of the Soviet Union's collapse, Kazakhstan inherited the remnants of one of the world's most contaminated landscapes: the Semipalatinsk Test Site, known locally as the Polygon. Resigned to dispossession, residents have chosen to remain on the abandoned nuclear test site, despite the isolation and the radioactive environment, rather than face marginalization or the rigour of a neoliberal world. *Atomic Collective* examines this nuclear legacy through a decade-long ethnographic examination of the village of Koian, situated on the border of the test site. Facing residual radiation all around them and isolation, Koianers persist, reshaping their pastoral existence among the ruins and scientific debates surrounding genetic damage.

Drawing on first-hand accounts and archival research, this book explores the resilience and everyday survival strategies of a community left behind to fend for itself in the shadow of nuclear testing. It offers a unique perspective on life in a nuclear zone and poses fundamental questions about human resilience and the impact of historical events on a collective identity. *Atomic Collective* sheds light on a community overlooked in the larger Cold War histories of atomic testing.

MAGDALENA E. STAWKOWSKI is a McCausland Faculty Fellow and an assistant professor in the Department of Anthropology at the University of South Carolina.

Atomic Collective

Radioactive Life in Kazakhstan

MAGDALENA E. STAWKOWSKI

UNIVERSITY OF TORONTO PRESS
Toronto Buffalo London

ISBN 978-1-4875-6029-4 (cloth)   ISBN 978-1-4875-6032-4 (EPUB)
ISBN 978-1-4875-6030-0 (paper)   ISBN 978-1-4875-6031-7 (PDF)

Library and Archives Canada Cataloguing in Publication

Title: Atomic collective : radioactive life in Kazakhstan / Magdalena E. Stawkowski.
Names: Stawkowski, Magdalena E., author.
Description: Includes bibliographical references and index.
Identifiers: Canadiana (print) 20240502426 | Canadiana (ebook) 20240503961 |
    ISBN 9781487560294 (cloth) | ISBN 9781487560300 (paper) | ISBN 9781487560324 (EPUB) |
    ISBN 9781487560317 (PDF)
Subjects: LCSH: Kazakhstan – Social life and customs – 21st century. | LCSH:
    Kazakhstan – Economic conditions – 21st century. | LCSH: Nuclear weapons –
    Testing – Social aspects – Kazakhstan. | LCSH: Nuclear weapons – Testing – Health
    aspects – Kazakhstan. | LCSH: Nuclear weapons – Testing –   Environmental
    aspects – Kazakhstan.
Classification: LCC DK906 .S73 2025 | DDC 958.45/08 – dc23

Cover design: Val Cooke
Cover images: (bottom) Cooling off in a test site lake at Semipalatinsk Nuclear Test Site,
June 2019 © Magdalena E. Stawkowski; (top) iStock.com/mas0380

We wish to acknowledge the land on which the University of Toronto Press
operates. This land is the traditional territory of the Wendat, the Anishnaabeg, the
Haudenosaunee, the Métis, and the Mississaugas of the Credit First Nation.

Publication of this book was made possible, in part, by a grant from the First Book
Subvention Program of the Association for Slavic, East European, and Eurasian Studies.

University of Toronto Press acknowledges the financial support of the Government of
Canada, the Canada Council for the Arts, and the Ontario Arts Council, an agency of
the Government of Ontario, for its publishing activities.

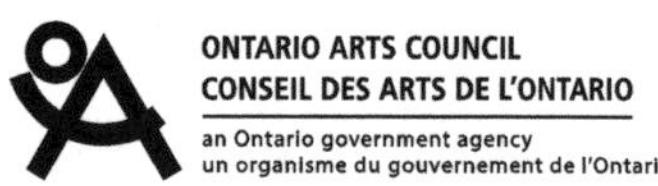

For my mother, Margaret, whose strong will is matched only by her fearlessness and indomitable spirit.

Contents

Illustrations

Foreword

To Live: Shadows of Fallout in Kazakhstan's Nuclear Test Site

Take a wild journey with anthropologist Dr. Magdalena Stawkowski across the windswept Kazakh steppes. See these steppes through the eyes of those who experienced the profound effects of Soviet atomic testing during the Cold War. Stawkowski takes both her academic colleagues and her civilian audience on a fascinating journey to the present-day location in Kazakhstan where the Soviet Union detonated hundreds of atomic bombs – both above ground and below ground – in Stalin's push to develop atomic weaponry after the United States dropped two atomic bombs on Japan. The testing site for these trials took place on what is now called the Semipalatinsk Test Site and its rural settlements positioned at its boundaries, a region that experienced more than 450 blasts. The ongoing effects on local populations are still being debated and uncovered, and it is this realization that sits at the centre of this ethnography: the people in this region are not waiting for the first or last word on expert debates. Their job is to live!

Stawkowski's fieldwork takes place in the quiet village of Koian (a pseudonym meaning "rabbit" in Kazakh), which the author visits periodically for more than a decade; she helps us understand the approach to the local way of life that Koianers have adopted. In August 1991, Kazakhstan's government shut down the nuclear site, and later that same year in December gained independence from the Soviet Union. Fast-forward to 2016, the Kazakh street artist Pasha Cas created a giant graffiti-like reproduction of Edvard Munch's *The Scream* on a leftover brick structure at the Semipalatinsk Test Site.[1] He renamed his political art piece *This Is Silence*, mirroring and yet diverging from Munch's original anxiety and despair. A well-known aspect of Munch's creation is that the artist lived next door to a psychiatric facility, where his sister was institutionalized. Placing this iconic replica (or perhaps, better said, reinterpretation) at Kazakhstan's nuclear site creates new meanings. While the country allows for a healthy anti-nuclear sensibility since independence, it seeks to leverage its natural resources and nuclear history to bolster its economy. Stawkowski's book provides voice and appreciation for a population still living at the margins of the test site and how they go about making a life while perfectly cognizant of *both* the imposing silence produced in the aftermath of the destruction that took place and the meaning of the scream, all of which encompass the fraught and anxious environment in which they navigate their own unique futures.

Many voices are represented in this lively ethnography, ranging from environmental activists to scientists of the post–Soviet era (who are the present-day keepers of the studies carried out in the region), alongside, of course, the people of Koian. Koianers who were children during this time or were told of the events and have come to consider this information much later are aware that they were made to be "experimental rabbits." Today, joint activism exists between the Nevada and Semipalatinsk test sites, both of which have seen populations living nearby with increased cancer rates and other health problems. And yet these health problems are still very much unsettled and a source of an ongoing public and scientific debate.

Koian may as well be on another planet, and we know well that the economic investment in Koianers and their surrounding communities will never obtain the hype associated with space exploration. While still on Earth, Koian has "no running water, no grocery store, no gas station, medical clinic, or even a school" (*Atomic Collective*, p. 11). There isn't even a road connecting Koian to the world outside. And yet, despite this neglect and the stigma of living on contaminated lands, the people of Koian seem to be at a place of deep peace with their fate. This stands in sharp relief to the possibilities of city life in Kazakhstan – also contaminated – and shows a reverence and depth of feeling for their ancestors buried on the lands they cherish and remain faithful to. In *Atomic Collective* we meet a representative of the environmental movement (Semyon) whose organization has been in favour of moving the villagers away from the test site and proposes securing the radioactive areas. Importantly, the communities they are aiming to protect resist such proposals and don't want to move. Stawkowski patiently explains why this is so.

The "people of the Polygon" – as they are often referred to outside Koian – are "shunned in cities, are abused in hospitals, and take jobs in mines where they are not permitted to measure radiation levels" (*Atomic Collective*, p. 18). Stawkowski explains that the people she came to know in Koian have "embraced" radiation and, in their consideration of alternative possibilities, have come to believe that their current option – of staying put where they are – is preferable to moving to the cities, being jammed into a small apartment in an urban setting, and still forced to breathe contaminated air. As the Koianer Burkut explains to Stawkowski, those who move to the cities survive only two years. "For many years we were exposed to radioactive fallout, and now we eat it. Slowly and quietly, our bodies got used to it. Why do you think people don't die in Koian, but only get a little sick ... Clean air is our death" (*Atomic Collective*, p. 56). Readers will get a sense of the vagaries of Stalinist excess and neglect: while this community benefited from agricultural extension, markets, and some aspects of collectivization, they were also "enduring bombs and serving as living medical experiments" (*Atomic Collective*, p. 23).

This book led me to wonder (again) about the multiple paths that led to the establishment of Institutional Review Boards, as well as how research was conducted during the Cold War (and we know that transgressions were common on both sides of that war). Stawkowski reports that until the "breakup of the Soviet Union in 1991, no official information or real medical assistance was offered to those examined by the dispensary's medical staff" (*Atomic Collective*, p. 36). Not all was grim. Koianers fondly remember the Soviet developmentalist period known as the Virgin Lands campaign that began in 1953, where Krushchev planned to boost the Soviet Union's agricultural production to alleviate food shortages and turned to northern Kazakhstan. Assessments of this campaign suggest that there was initial short-term success, with increased production and the alleviation of food shortages from 1954 to 1960. But by the early 1960s, productivity significantly declined and never quite recovered. While many Koianers remember the Virgin Lands campaign positively, as with the long-standing critiques of the Green Revolution in Mexico and other regions of the Global South, much of the land apportioned to the Virgin Lands campaign and its success was eventually understood to be temporary and to have contributed to soil erosion and deleterious ecological conditions because of the monocultural intensity of the campaign. By the early 1960s, the campaign was deemed an unmitigated disaster.

So, despite the voluminous academic literature deeming both the nuclear testing and the Virgin Lands campaign to have caused tandem ecological disasters in the region, Koianers display a curiously different stance. For them, it is their land, their home, and the place of their ancestors. Their quest is to survive whatever catastrophes are sent their way. Leaving is simply unthinkable.

There is, too, a curious detail noted by Koianers themselves. Apparently, after each nuclear test, Soviet commanders would give "150 grams of vodka" to the soldiers. This vodka-induced defence against nuclear things has been described in Svetlana Alexievich's[2] account of the catastrophic nuclear meltdown at Chornobyl (Chernobyl) in 1986, when vodka became the currency for negotiations among parties dealing with the evacuation and clean-up of the area. While Chornobyl (Chernobyl) became better known than the events in Kazakhstan, the soldiers involved in cleaning up this nuclear disaster became known as Chornobylites. This term referred to them as if they were a separate category of humans, pointing to their potential biological and genetic damage. Koianers learned about their own situation in the late 1980s when the Nevada-Semipalatinsk anti-nuclear movement made this information publicly available. Also, on the other side of the world, the *Bulletin of the Atomic Scientists* let it be known in 1997 that the Atomic Energy Commission – among other US government entities – was negligent in warning populations of contamination to milk in regions near the Nevada nuclear test site. The data became known only in a 1997 National Cancer Institute report that children were exposed to more radiation than was initially reported,[3] and much of this exposure came through drinking contaminated milk. Apparently, now, public documents show that in one 1956 detonation in Kazakhstan, more than six hundred people ended up in the hospital for radiation sickness and that the Soviets knew about these health effects (*Atomic Collective*, p. 156n65) but did not act to competently prevent them. And yet despite all of this bad faith activity, many Koianers often consider the Soviet era in a positive light, especially when compared with the uncertainty of the post-Soviet period.

In the more recent renderings of the Semipalatinsk Test Site, the Kazakh government's Institute of Radiation Safety and Ecology, the newest version of what was once a part of the many secret Soviet cities devoted to nuclear weaponry, is now located in the city of Kurchatov and is tasked with researching the test site and ensuring safe conditions. Stawkowski notes ironically that some of their efforts are devoted to expanding its nuclear energy program, extracting uranium for Western markets, and most bizarrely, even designing programs and initiatives to combat what is understood as "radiophobia." Radiophobia seems to provide an ideological framework to dismiss and discredit legitimate concerns about radiation contamination and to forward national programs with market profitability. Some other factions in the country have alternatively tried to prove that Koianers and others like them are by now biologically damaged or compromised, generating a kind of voyeuristic medical interest in the people living at the site.

In the meantime, too, the regional shift from a planned to a market economy meant that Koianers faced many challenges. The change meant that their *sovkhoz* (state-owned farm) went bankrupt and much of the essential infrastructure was left to decay. Despite the economic catastrophe, Koianers succeeded in helping one another survive these shifts in resources, infrastructure, and mindset. While debates and disagreements are taking place, Koianers are most actively living their lives, navigating between the extreme positions of believing that nothing much has happened to them and that it is possible that something quite serious has happened to them. Rather than seeing themselves as genetic mutants, they view themselves instead as survivors of evolutionary advance, proposing that everyone is a "little bit sick." According to Stawkowski, the people of Koian prefer to live *"sami po sebe,"* that is "on their own and keeping to themselves" (*Atomic Collective*, p. 74). Some of this is simply due to neglect under the market economy but is also the result of Koian's nuclear history. And while one might have hoped for a more creative gender configuration of labour in their resistance to the futures presented to them by others and in their quest to be "on their own," Stawkowski tells us that new societal pressures have emerged: bride abduction has come back into fashion (even in places where it never existed), a sign that Koianer resistance to the will of others might also produce some unexpected gender distinctions.

In *Atomic Collective*, we learn that with all that has happened in Kazakhstan and in the region of the test site, no state organization is overseeing or regulating the radiation levels of food products (*Atomic Collective*, p. 84). In this context, Stawkowski again reminds us, Koianers "cheerfully fend for themselves" (*Atomic Collective*, p. 96). And when they are treated by the author to a few days of high-class spa treatment in an expensive resort, they manage to "have a tremendous amount of fun" even while being seen in that context as country bumpkins by the Russian-speaking Kazakhs. We later learn that they also take pleasure in seeing themselves as superior to Kazakhstani Mongolians who migrate to Kazakhstan.

Perhaps the most obvious bad-faith pursuit that we see throughout the book is the misguided use of vodka to protect against radiation. While the rest of the world was cheerfully believing that red wine in moderate amounts helped to fend off heart disease and high cholesterol,[4] in Kazakhstan, vodka has been promoted as the magic tonic to ward off radiation exposure. According to Stawkowski, there are most likely additional cancers and other health issues that require explanation: the life expectancy around the Polygon is seven years less than the rest of Kazakhstan.

Some might ask, well then, what is to be done? The answer, it seems, is to let these people live as they want. Stawkowski is not advocating for neglect. Private enterprise is staking claims to potential profits on the Polygon, and Koianers must deal with some competition for the land they inhabit. Indeed, I came away from this captivating book feeling some deep kindred spirit with Koianers and their sense of collective life. I sympathized with their long history and attempts to continue to live, collectively, as they wish despite the follies of the nuclear era and despite the intensifying neoliberal tendencies of the Kazakh state. Stawkowski rightly presents a portrait of a proud people who are determined to set the conditions of their own futures.

Donna M. Goldstein, Professor of Anthropology

Acknowledgments

I extend my deepest gratitude to the proud people of Koian, who welcomed me into their midst, shared their lives with me, and showed me a world I otherwise would never have known. Their circumstances are difficult. Living with them, I learned what it means to persevere in the face of a catastrophe and to have the profound capacity to discover joy in the most unlikely of places, like a sudden crop of wild strawberries, even if found on a nuclear test site. Without their kindness and wisdom to guide me through a vast expanse of the Kazakh steppe (which often kept me out of harm's way or got my car out of deep mud), there would be no book to read. Although most names and locales that appear in this book have been altered, I am indebted to so many friends and comrades from villages dotting the nuclear test site, as well as the cities of Kurchatov, Karaganda, Semey, Pavlodar, Astana, Almaty, and many others, who graciously shared their insights with me, be it through casual conversations, during interviews, or at summer get-togethers. Their stories have made a permanent imprint on my life, and I find myself always eager to return.

In Kazakhstan, there are many individuals whose advice and support with the research, in their archives of faded Soviet newspapers, their photographs of anti-nuclear demonstrations, and their experience in the precarious world of public policy, gave direction to this work. I could never thank enough Dima and Yulia, Dana, Kaisha, Alexander, Naila, as well as Yuliya, Irina, Konstantin, Elena, Anna, Dimitry, Sasha, Ludmila, Olga, Vadim, Nadezhda, Alina, Oleg, Anton, Sergey, Vladimir, Ivan, Nina, Wanda, Denis, and countless others who helped and advised on this project.

It has been a long road, all tired metaphors aside. In summer 2009, I began the initial stages of a research project that would eventually lead me to Koian. This book began with preliminary fieldwork when I was a graduate student at the University of Colorado, Boulder (CU-Boulder). Throughout the early phases and my growing stack of field journals, I was fortunate to have financial support from various grants and fellowships, including those from the Department of Anthropology at CU-Boulder, the Goldstein Altman Grant, the Albert E. Smith Fund for the New Nuclear Age, the National Science Foundation Research Experiences for Graduates (NSF REG), and the Center to Advance Research and Teaching in the Social Sciences (CARTSS). Subsequent phases of fieldwork and dissertation writing were generously supported by organizations such as the Social Science Research Council Eurasia Program Dissertation Development Award Fellowship, the International Research & Exchanges Board's Individual Advanced Research Opportunities Program (IREX IARO), the University of Colorado Boulder Graduate School Dissertation Completion Fellowship, and the P.E.O. Scholar Award.

During my years at CU-Boulder, both as a master's and a PhD student, and beyond, I have had the privilege and the best fortune to work with an exceptional adviser, mentor, and now a dear friend, Donna Goldstein. Her brilliance as an anthropologist notwithstanding, her guidance, patience, and encouragement were instrumental in shaping me into a better scholar, colleague, and individual. Over the years, she has challenged me to think deeply about the world around us and ask important questions with empathy and compassion. Our exchanges over that time and the always fascinating and complex collaborative projects we embark on were (and remain), my grounding as an anthropologist in her footsteps. As I reflect on it now (and I'm certain she'd laugh), I realize that without her, I would never be writing acknowledgments to an ethnography. I am endlessly grateful for her sharp mind and invaluable comments on both my dissertation and the entire draft of this book, along with her infectious humour and unwavering support during life's trials and tribulations. Thank you for everything.

CU-Boulder was my rock. I benefited immeasurably from mentors and colleagues there. I am deeply appreciative to Kira Hall for her intellectual support and encouragement. Many thanks also to Carla Jones for believing in this project and allotting generous amounts of time to help me see it through, as well as Jerry Peterson, Bryan Taylor, Bert Covert, Tim Oakes, Paul Shankman, Dennis McGilvray, and Carole McGranahan. Len Ackland (and his wonderful partner, Carol) helped me confront the complexities and barriers of radiation science, as well as shared with me his prolific research and knowledge of Rocky Flats. Through Len, I was fortunate to meet LeRoy Moore from the Rocky Mountain Peace and Justice Center. Others at CU-Boulder that I extend thanks to include my mentors Mark Leiderman, Tatiana Mikhailova, and Padraic Kenney, all of whom have left Boulder for other academic settings, and who provided me with a solid introduction to Soviet and post-Soviet scholarship. Without CU-Boulder, I'd never have met the wonderful scholars, now colleagues, from other institutions: Longina Jakubowska, Anton Blok, Laurence Carucci, Barbara Rose Johnston, and Eva Castringius. Susanne Bauer helped me to think through the complex research on human radiation exposure impacts, especially in Soviet and post-Soviet contexts.

An amazing circle of friends in graduate school is priceless. My heartfelt gratitude extends to Jessica Hedgepeth Balkin for her unwavering friendship, and to Christopher Morris, Meryleen Mena, Willi Lempert, Lindsay Ofrias, James Dubendorf, Marnie Thomson, Kate Fischer, Jamie Forde, Anna Hermann, Bridget Hanna, and James Millette. A special thank you is reserved for Katy Putsavage, whose daring and endless support led her to fly to the snow-covered steppes of Kazakhstan in December to keep me company. (That was a great New Year's in Almaty!).

Writing is a lifelong journey. I am indebted to Kate Brown for her guidance and suggestions on how to transform a dissertation into a book, especially how to think in terms of narrative arcs and to avoid "purple prose." Her work is an inspiration to confront tough topics and write about them without hubris but never lacking confidence. Many thanks go to Lynne Viola and her fabulous graduate student reading group at the University of Toronto, and the snowy nights, which encouraged intellectual rigour and stimulated great conversations. Thank you very much to Natalie Koch for sharing her work with me. Our regular check-in phone calls over the years have sustained me through the writing process. I also want to express my gratitude to Robert Borofsky, who regularly called to check in on me and encouraged me to keep going.

Leaving CU-Boulder, my interest in all things nuclear took many turns. In 2013, I joined Wilson Center's the Nuclear Proliferation International History Project's Nuclear Boot Camp in Allumiere, Italy. This was a ten-day immersion program focused on nuclear history, from the Manhattan Project and arms control to nuclear non-proliferation and other nuclear-related topics at an utterly fascinating decommissioned Italian Air Force Base (which once served as a pivotal link in NATO communications network). With the quaint dormitory atop a steep road and lively dinners in the town below, I was surrounded by experts in the field who helped refine my thinking about the complex legacies of our nuclear age. I am especially grateful to Martin Sherwin (who left this world too soon), Leopoldo Nutti, Christian Ostermann, Emma Rosengren, Joseph Pilat, Marilena Gala, Robynne Mellor, Niccolò Petrelli, and Flavia Gasbarri, as well as Rabia Akhtar, and Jayita Sarkar, among many others.

I would like to extend a special thank you to David Holloway, a prominent expert on the history of Soviet nuclear weapons development. I am so grateful for his kindness. During my time as a Stanton Nuclear Security Postdoctoral Fellow and the MacArthur Nuclear Security Postdoctoral Fellowship at the Center for International Security and Cooperation (CISAC) at Stanford University, David was the best mentor one could ask for. He shared his insights with me on how to write a compelling book, graciously, and helped me to think about the Soviet atomic bomb project in a new light.

Stanford University was a whole world of great support. I am especially grateful to Sig Hecker, who has done impactful non-proliferation work in Kazakhstan, as well as Lynn Eden, Rodney Ewing, Scott Sagan, Gil-li Vardi, and Brad Roberts. A small group of dear friends and colleagues at CISAC, Jackie Kerr, Elaine Korzak, Edward Geist, James Cameron, Christopher Lawrence, and Andreas Kuehn, made life superbly entertaining and deeply intellectual. I thank Amir Weiner. In many ways, we share parallel life trajectories marked by hardship that extend to the types of scholarship we do. Additionally, his fondness for the titles of my articles has always been a source of laughter and insightful conversations, especially with the participants of the Kruzhok reading group he directed at the time. Thank you to Koyko Sato and Mark Gardiner for their friendship and intellectual community. Fragments of this book were first written in a beautiful home, just down the road in Los Altos. Thank you to Paul Mockapetris and his family for kindly offering that space of rose gardens and fruit trees, where I found inspiration and a peaceful space to write.

As a postdoctoral and visiting scholar at North Carolina State University and the University of North Carolina Chapel Hill, I am fortunate to have received the valuable comments and suggestions on early drafts of an article, parts of which appear in this book, from Molly Mullin and Nora Haenn. Thanks also to Shea McManus, Raja Abillama, and Vasilina Orlova for their support and wonderfully refreshing conversations about all sorts of things.

At my new home in the Palmetto State, I am part of a wonderfully supportive and collaborative anthropology department at the University of South Carolina. My colleagues, many of whom are now good friends, have been stellar. In particular, I want to thank my amazing current chair, Jennifer Reynolds, and the always encouraging Marc

Moskowitz, whose support, big and small, is much appreciated. They have been generous with their time and protected mine by giving me the space to finish this book. Both also provided insightful comments and offered editing suggestions on the final draft of the introduction. I would also like to thank Monica Barra for her companionship and valuable feedback during the many conversations we've had over dinners. Thanks also to David Simmons, Kim Simmons, Terrance Weik, Carlina de la Cova, John Doering-White, Chelsea Fisher, Jelena Jankovic-Rankovic, and Joanna Casey, as well as colleagues who have left the department for other academic settings, Sharon DeWitte, Sherina Feliciano-Santos, and Courtney Lewis. I extend my heartfelt gratitude to Drucilla Barker who I miss sincerely. May you rest in power, dear friend.

Elsewhere at the University of South Carolina, special thanks go to the Critical Ecologies Lab of geographers, historians, and anthropologists working at the intersection of science and technology studies to address pressing environmental issues. It is unlike any other group I've ever known. Thanks Jessica Barnes, David Kneas, Meredith DeBoom, Dean Hardy, Conor Harrison, Joshua Grace, and Thomas Lekan for the terrifically intellectual workshop space. To Timothy Mousseau, thank you for deepening my understanding of radiation effects on plants and animals (I now know way too much about grasshoppers) and for travelling with me to Kazakhstan in summer 2023 to start a new and exciting project that was years in the making.

The first draft of this book began to take shape in January 2020, in a small flat in Copenhagen. Support for this work and research trips to Kazakhstan in 2019 and 2023 were made possible through generous funding from the Danish Council for Independent Research, in collaboration with colleagues from the Danish Institute for International Studies on a project titled Radioactive Ruins: Security in the Age of the Anthropocene. I am indebted to the Wenner-Gren Foundation Hunt Postdoctoral Fellowship, as well, which allowed me to dedicate a full year to writing without teaching obligations.

As the COVID-19 pandemic unfolded in March 2020, Denmark closed its borders. Consequently, I remained there until mid-June. I am grateful to the Danish Institute for International Studies for welcoming me and for the companionship and support of colleagues and friends, Rens van Munster, and graduate student (at the time), Lis Kaiser. With offices, academic institutions, and restaurants on lockdown, we spent many hours in Copenhagen's verdant city parks, contemplating the sociocultural legacies of nuclear testing and the lives of people who experienced the effects of radioactive fallout first-hand and those who came after. I am indebted to Rens and Lis for their keen insights that helped refine some of the ideas I present in this book. I would also like to thank my assistant, Maksat Zhanibek, for his invaluable help in the archives during the final year of the project. His expertise and dedication have been a great support, both in wrapping up this work and in getting my new project underway.

I am profoundly grateful for the support of my incredible colleague and friend Joanna Mishtal. She spent several days at my house in Columbia, South Carolina, meticulously reviewing the final draft of the entire manuscript, providing insightful comments and tirelessly substantive points throughout. Her unparalleled attention to detail, thorough feedback, and intellectual rigour helped improve this book. Thank you for our wonderful conversations over the years and advice on all matters academic and not. Your keen observations about the world, coupled with a great sense of humour, are always appreciated. Thank you also to Marc Elie who provided feedback on the historical chapter, as well as Paul Josephson who regularly shared his work with me and periodically checked in on my progress from afar.

This book would certainly not be the same without the unwavering support of my amazing friend, colleague, and partner, Robert Kopack. He accompanied me on several trips to Kazakhstan while doing his own research there. Throughout my project and the revisions of this draft, he provided sound guidance, constructive feedback, and editorial advice with care. His vast knowledge of Kazakhstan's Soviet-era clandestine military cities and the many conversations over the years we've had about them brought into sharper focus the various historical, social, political, and economic consequences of their development on the places and people that once sustained them. Robert's support during moments of personal tragedy that punctuated my research and early stages of writing has been a lifeline for me. It was in these moments that his generosity and encouragement pushed me over the finish line. I am forever grateful.

I also consider myself incredibly fortunate to have found an editor, Olson Pook, who was willing to embark on this writing journey with me. I am thankful to him for being not only a meticulous editor but also a kind and patient person. He helped to refine my argument and insisted I stay true to my convictions and to always consider my audience. I am deeply grateful for his unwavering support.

Sincere thank you to the University of Toronto Press and particularly to Stephen Shapiro, who believed in this project from the start. Stephen's dedication and guidance to seeing this book come to fruition cannot be overstated. I am immensely privileged to have had an opportunity to work with such an incredible editor whose support and feedback made the publishing process easier to navigate. I am deeply appreciative of Leah Connor for overseeing the production process of this book. Leah's support and dedication meant that everything came together smoothly. Thank you. Many thanks also to Stephanie Mazza and Vesna Micic for their invaluable support with the book. My sincere gratitude also goes to Dawn Hunter, my copy editor, for her meticulous attention to detail and suggestions that have greatly improved the clarity of this book. I also want to extend many thanks to Sergey Lobachev, my indexer, for crafting a comprehensive and accessible index that has made this book much easier to navigate for readers. Many thanks also to the anonymous reviewers for their constructive comments. A special thanks to Harris Bienn for his exceptional work in crafting the maps for this book. Publication of this book was made possible, in part, by a grant from the First Book Subvention Program of the Association for Slavic, East European, and Eurasian Studies. I also received support from the University of South Carolina College of Arts and Sciences Book Manuscript Finalization Support Initiative.

I want to extend my appreciation to additional friends and colleagues unmentioned up to this point, such as my Colorado intellectual community, including Grace Hood, Priscilla Craven, Mary Louise Edwards, and Vince Darcangelo. Thank you also to Maxime Polleri, Jacob Hamblin, Melanie Arndt, Anna Weichselbraun, Vincent Ialenti, Livia Monnet, Zachary Androus, Daniel Renfrew, Tatiana Chudakova, and Claudia Heinermann. Thanks also to Sarah Putsavage for supporting my P.E.O. Scholar Award.

Finally, I want to express my gratitude to my family, who were there throughout. I am especially forever grateful to my amazing mother, Margaret (Małgorzata), for always believing in me and teaching me to never give up. Her strength and love of life, despite it all, gave meaning to mine. I also extend a great big hug and gratitude to my nephew, Aleksander, who made my life a little brighter, as well as to Tomasz Mikulski, for giving me a place in Poland to unwind after travelling to Kazakhstan. My artist sister, Ala, if only life were different. Thank you also to my aunt Marlena Szydelski for good company and Polish dinners, as well as my uncle Jerry and cousins Ola (Alexandra) and Matt. My utterly spoiled pups, Babette and Yola, for always keeping me company and making writing a much happier affair. And to all acquaintances I may have forgotten – thank you.

A note on chapters. Certain portions of this book were published in article form. Chapter 2, titled "'Clean Air Is Our Death': Debates about Genetic Mutation," is based on two separate articles: "'I Am a

Radioactive Mutant': Emergent Biological Subjectivities at Kazakhstan's Semipalatinsk Nuclear Test Site," published in *American Ethnologist* in 2016, and "Radiophobia Had to Be Reinvented," which appeared in the journal of *Culture, Theory and Critique* in 2017. Additionally, early attempts to develop my arguments and some of the stories presented in this book appeared in condensed form in my article "Life on an Atomic Collective: The Post-Soviet Retreat of the State in Rural Kazakhstan," which was published in the journal *Études Rurales* in 2017.

This book uses the American Library Association and Library of Congress (ALA-LC) transliteration. It faithfully represents each Cyrillic letter in Latin script, ensuring that Russian and Kazakh terms retain their meaning. The only exception is "Polygon," which I use instead of the transliterated "Poligon" because "Polygon" is commonly used in popular media and scientific literature.

ATOMIC COLLECTIVE

Introduction: "Discovering" Koian

Like it or not,
Your genes have a political past,
Your skin a political cast,
Your eyes a political aspect.
What you say has a resonance;
what you are silent about is telling.
Either way, it's political.
Even when you head for the hills
you're taking political steps
on political ground.

– Wisława Szymborska, Children of Our Era

It's mid-June 2019. The spring rains have ended, and the silent heat fills the wide blue sky. What was knee-deep mud is again a fine powder-dust. The air conditioner in the car is broken, but the windows are up. The steppe path has turned into a river of the stuff and it's everywhere – on the steering wheel, the dashboard, the windows, and the floor. It even sticks to the stuffy suits we're wearing, which damp with sweat feel like a thin layer of plaster. In the distance, we see clouds of dust forming a trail in the sky outlining the path of an oncoming car. When it arrives, the driver casually leans out of the window and asks, "How far to Koian?" "About three hours, maybe more, but watch out for the muddy creek; someone got stuck there earlier," I say through a barely cracked window before bidding them farewell.

It feels strange to pass cars on these roads. We are in fully enclosed and hermetically sealed disposable Tyvek hazmat suits, sweating profusely underneath their impermeable layers, while every car we pass cruises by blasting Europop music with the windows down and the occupants unmasked. We must look completely insane or alien or both – visitors from a parallel universe.

The irony of the situation is not lost on me; out here there really are parallel universes. We are in northeast Kazakhstan, inside the perimeter of the Semipalatinsk Test Site, also known locally as the "Polygon" (which is a Russian word for any military firing range). It's where the Soviet Union tested more than 450 nuclear bombs over a forty-year period, unleashing the power of more than twenty-five hundred Hiroshima-sized bombs on a territory the size of New Jersey, only to abandon it after 1991 as decrepit defence infrastructure.

My assistant, Olek, half-jokingly says we are in a "national park" – what he calls "our own savannah: pure nature and wild animals." He's in IT and works with an ecological research centre back in Karaganda, hundreds of kilometres and a world away from where we are. We've seen plenty of *argali* (wild mountain sheep), foxes, ground squirrels, rabbits, hawks, and even a wolf along the way. The vast expanses of grassland bring to mind parts of sub-Saharan Africa or the Great Plains in the United States. For Olek, this is a chance to get out of the city for a few days. But for me, the people we passed earlier, and the residents who live in this region, this place is a *shortcut*. Driving through the Polygon's nearly seven thousand square miles (about eighteen thousand square kilometres) is a way to save time. If you're lucky, travelling around the perimeter of the nuclear zone from Koian – a windswept village on the western border of the site – to Semey on the eastern border will take a little over twenty-four hours. If you're willing to enter the Polygon and successfully cross it in a straight line, it takes barely half a day.

Of course, few shortcuts in Kazakhstan are trickier to navigate than the Polygon and the regions around it. For hundreds of kilometres, it's an open steppe sliced by a confusing patchwork of dirt roads that seem to go everywhere and nowhere. These trails cross over towering humps, skitter down into trenches of stony streams and up again to face wide-open fields of thigh-high grass. It took me months to figure out how to find Koian on my own, how to see with new eyes a practically non-existent sandy path through the flat fields as it curves this way and that, sometimes running along sagging lines of utility poles, then away from them "up and over the grey hill" and then "taking a left after the field for horses."

Despite spending almost a decade engaged in ethnographic research in Koian, I had never cut across the entire nuclear test site before. Getting through without a guide, GPS, or the mental imprint of dozens of prior trips would be nigh impossible; there are few remaining signs

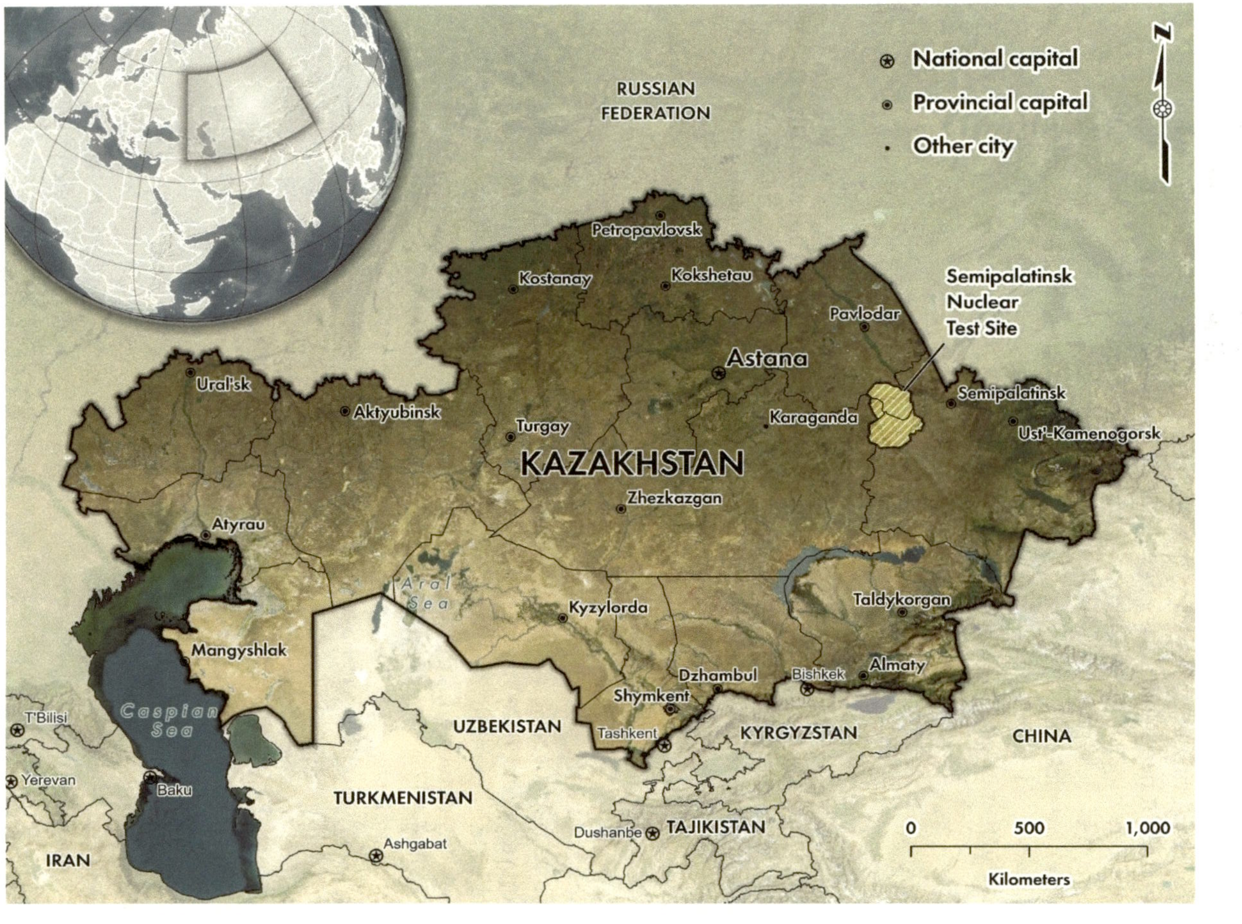

Map 1. Kazakhstan

or fences from the Soviet era directing traffic. Thankfully, I have Olek. He's done this trip a dozen times with the research centre he works for. For my part, I've embraced the first rule of travelling in and around the Polygon: bring extras of everything. Our Jeep Cherokee is packed with stuff we'll need should we get stuck or break down: two twenty-litre canisters of gasoline we bartered in Koian, a spare tyre, shovel, flashlight, a bicycle pump, several lengths of rope, and two ten-litre jugs of water we picked up days earlier in Karaganda. Tursynbek and Altynai, my adopted family back in Koian, are awaiting my check-in once I arrive in Semey or they'll come looking for us.

Driving through what should be an "exclusion zone" isn't something that I just hadn't gotten around to – far from it. I had intentionally avoided crossing the Polygon. Most often I stayed in Koian, aside from a few short trips darting in and out of the test site for supplies or to satisfy my curiosity about this or that point. Why anyone would choose to pass over the X found on Google Maps where hundreds of nuclear detonations had been staged mystified me. Few areas of the world are as polluted as the Polygon. This is where the swelling mushroom-like clouds and fiery red, orange, and white rings changed the Kazakh plains into an atomic no-man's-land in 1949, marking the arrival of the Anthropocene – the new geologic epoch of human-caused environmental transformation.[1] The massive radioactive plumes from these explosions scattered radiation and ash far and wide across the Polygon, and much of this land remains scorched by fallout that no one can see, hear, smell, or taste.

I likely would never have taken this trip had it not been for the vagaries of ethnographic research. Interviews are often not always planned well in advance, and a sudden opening left me scrambling to get to Semey's Scientific Research Institute for Radiation Medicine and Ecology with less than a week left on my visa. The only choice I had to make the interviews on time was to take the shortcut.

Back in Koian, people thought I was paranoid. Wearing the hazmat suit was proof. "Did you forget you're *used* to radiation?" Tursynbek laughed. Most people in this depopulated region don't worry about it. But try as I might, I can't unlearn what I've read in scientific journals about the health effects of acute and low-dose exposure to ionizing radiation. We not only pass other cars bouncing through the area with their windows down but also see shepherds on horseback leading

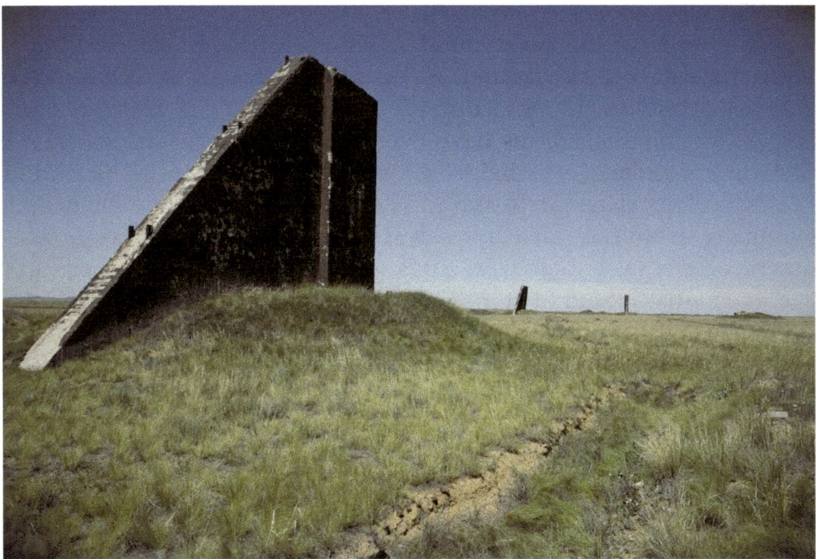

Figure I.1. *Concrete Geese*. Remnants of concrete structures once filled with sensors to measure the force of a nuclear blast. Locals call them "geese." They extend in a straight line from the above-ground test epicentre and resemble giant goose necks emerging from a sea of green steppe grass.

flocks of sheep or goats to watering holes and watch as large and jostling Soviet-era Kamaz trucks brimming with payloads of coal or other substances depart mines in the area. The setting for all this myriad activity is punctuated by rows of towering concrete structures built to photograph and measure atomic blasts during the Cold War. Passing by, I can see trenches for electrical wires and pipes connecting the towers having been dug up and scavenged, with the remnants of barbed wire fencing sitting coiled off to the side.

In our white Tyvek coveralls, face masks, goggles, latex gloves, and knee-high rubber boots, it's an understatement to say that Olek and I stand out in this environment. I am convinced the gear will save us, keeping the radioactive dust from getting on our skin and into our lungs. Even though it won't entirely protect us from the invisible radiation – for that you need a shield six feet (about two metres) thick made of concrete or one foot (thirty centimetres) of lead – I made sure to bring my handheld Geiger counter and a set of extra batteries. Invented at the dawn of the nuclear age to detect ambient radiation in soil and rock or anything else, it's a useful tool to have. At the very least, the instrument will help us avoid the worst of the radiation – or so I hope.

As strange as it may sound, in Kazakhstan best practices do exist with regard to how to move through a nuclear test site. State agencies and environmental groups have even developed guidelines. When I first came to Koian, I even helped circulate informative pamphlets from Olek's ecological research centre. They contained cartoon characters telling drivers to keep away from dust plumes, not to stop to fix broken-down vehicles (as if there were a bus service that would pick them up), and even what I thought at the time was absurd advice, like not to picnic or swim in the craters formed by the explosions while on site.

Other materials distributed to people living in and around the Polygon advise against hunting animals for eating, gathering hay, or collecting metal. But by now I'm not surprised when Olek stops at a spot familiar to him to cool off. He happily removes his hazmat suit and dives into a deep-blue lake with a sandy beach on the other side, not unlike those found at a tropical resort.

Having spent years working in and around the Polygon, what struck me on this trip was that there weren't *more* people at the lake jumping in with him. He whoops and hollers as he climbs up a ladder and onto a cement diving dock built who knows how long ago, the sounds echoing against the rock-strewn walls of the lake. Village residents, scientists, and environmental activists have all told me about how popular these lakes are with their diving boards and makeshift volleyball courts. Regardless of the risks, people keep coming, and the ground is littered with cigarette butts, beer cans, and empty tins. The hot air whips the sand in all directions, and I can imagine the visitors who keep coming saying it's the perfect place to take a dip.

According to my Geiger counter, the lake itself technically isn't a radioactive hotspot despite many others right nearby. This is surprising as I'm quite literally standing on ground zero of the *Opytnoe Pole* (Experimental Field) – the location where every above-ground test was conducted. The lake itself resides inside a bowl-shaped crater punched into the steppe floor from an underground test. On the cement dock overlooking the water, I take in this tropical disaster-scape. Seeing it first-hand reinforced my view that the pamphlets, like the "duck and cover" exercises of the 1950s, are completely detached from the lived reality of those Kazakhs who populate the region.

It's not against the law to enter the Polygon or to work here; it's an open range with few signs that warn of danger. Nor is it possible to avoid the dust plumes – or convince Olek (who I thought should know better) not to take a dip on a scorching summer day. As we wound our

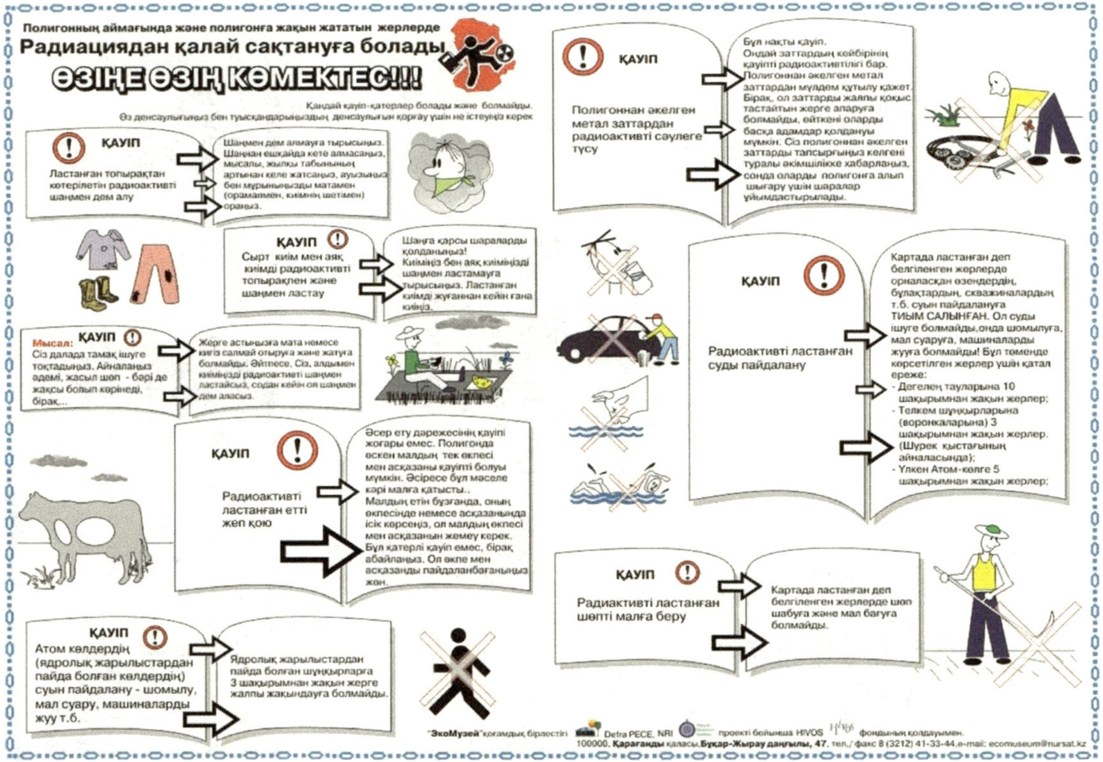

Figure I.2. *Radiation Safety Pamphlet*. A radiation safety pamphlet advising against various activities on the Polygon. It warns people not to drink milk from cows grazing on the site, picnic, cut grass, swim in lakes, wash cars, or harvest hay. The pamphlet also warns that animals should not drink water from the site and people should avoid walking there. Written in Kazakh, it emphasizes clothing contamination and advises against bringing contaminated clothes into the house.

way over the dirt paths, I was reminded of the fact that people have always lived inside the perimeter of the Polygon. Old crosses and crescent moons marked cemeteries from long ago, and I had even learned to identify abandoned winter pastures by the remains of stone and concrete buildings – as if people picked up the bricks and left with their radioactive homes in tow.

Olek finishes off his swim and I am happy to leave the lake behind and get back on the road. The dusty trail becomes more compacted but is simultaneously horribly potholed, and we have to ease our way over ditches of baked mud or go around them, speeding up whenever we can to make up for lost time. We finally roll onto pavement that looks suspiciously like a concrete airstrip. Two horses, one brown and the other grey, rub their heads on a signpost that reads in Russian and Kazakh: Attention! Hunting Without a Permit Is Prohibited! Such signs are common on the edges of the Polygon, alerting us to the fact that we have made the crossing. There are massed outlines of animal herds on the steppe casting long shadows, and I see little streams of chimney smoke in the distance. Just beyond is Kurchatov, the former secret city and administrative centre of the Soviet-era nuclear bomb project. It is connected by a meandering ribbon of asphalt that we will take to Semey, where I will meet with doctors, epidemiologists, and other scientists. Their predecessors kept detailed secret notes about the effects of radiation on the human body during the Cold War, housed in a secret clinic and kept from the people who lived in and around the Polygon, including the families in Koian whom I've come to know.

The lands in and around the Polygon are historically Kazakh and since the mid-twentieth century have been linked to monumental Soviet projects. All the villages contiguous with the test site and the homesteads inside the grounds were developed as part of a Soviet campaign to transform the people into proper communists and the open fields into vast farmlands. In these industrial-scale enterprises, men, women, and children learned to raise thousands of animals – sheep, goats, cows, and horses – while harvesting crops for Russians living thousands of kilometres away in cities. As newly designated citizens of the Soviet Union, they were provided housing, employment, and social welfare amid the liberally applied (since the late 1970s) layers of toxic fertilizers, pesticides, and herbicides while, one after another, nuclear bombs spewed radiation on them. For forty years, Soviet authorities made sure residents were kept in the dark, unaware of the danger posed by radiation. The testing regime itself was as clandestine as any in the world at the time.[2] Villagers in Koian and others like them told me about that they didn't suspect a thing, except when a neighbour got unexpectedly sick and quickly died or the occasional child was born with congenital anomalies, missing arms or legs, or with their organs inside out. Scientists working for the Soviet Ministry of Health would chalk up such events to an "unsanitary lifestyle" while busily collecting blood samples and other data on the effects of radiation exposure on the human body.[3] Just like nuclear testing, the data were a protected state secret until the late 1980s, some of it housed in a formerly secret clinic in Semey.

Today, thousands of people still live in and around the Polygon, an economically depressed region inhabited mostly by ethnic Kazakhs. More than one million people are officially recognized by the Kazakh state as victims of nuclear testing.[4] Koian residents belong to a "minimal-risk category" and are entitled to a one-time, lump-sum payment equalling about 50 USD.[5] Yet in the villages that dot the landscape, people live predominantly off the land and do not "observe" the Polygon border, which is poorly marked. Accessible to anyone who wishes to enter, there remain several protected areas where fissile materials like plutonium and highly enriched uranium could have been scavenged in the past.[6] But the perimeter of the site lacks physical borders of any kind and few signs point to radiation danger.

The lack of warning is not due to a lack of risk. The village of Koian, for example, is only a few kilometres from three craters caused by underground nuclear blasts. Some of these events were so-called "emergency situations," in which high concentrations of radioactive caesium, strontium, and americium were inadvertently vented into the environment at a distance of "several kilometers."[7] Koian is also only a short distance from Opytnoe Pole (ground zero) where I travelled with Olek. The 116 above-ground tests held there were primarily responsible for contaminating much of the Polygon as well as regions located hundreds of kilometres away, severely impacting human health as a result.[8] In areas as close as a kilometre and a half from the village, radiation levels are one hundred times higher than what is considered normal background levels. Just outside of the village, my Geiger counter registered 0.700 milliRem/hr –enough radiation to receive the average yearly dose in only five weeks.[9]

Like many isolated settlements, Koian is mostly abandoned, but around fifty people continue to live there, going on with their lives among the ruins that surround them. There is no running water, no grocery store, no gas station, medical clinic, or even a school. Koian doesn't have a *road*. People live in little single-storey whitewashed houses with blue (these days sometimes teal) trim next to rickety barns that somehow continue to stand under mountains of drying hay. Some buildings are no more than rubble heaps, disassembled for saleable brick, windows, and wiring. Many telephone poles long ago became firewood that blackened the walls of poorly ventilated homes. Koianers stock plenty of candles, have mountains of dung and truck loads of coal to burn for heat, and speak mostly Kazakh to each other, with the occasional Russian word thrown in. People raise animals – cows, horses, goats, and sheep – and travel by car or sometimes on foot for two-week shifts at whatever mine is hiring cheap labour. Barter has mostly replaced monetary exchange. And just over a small hill, where people frequently go to retrieve a loose horse, several bomb craters – themselves no more remarkable than odd mounds of dirt from a distance – gather water.[10]

This book is a tale of everyday life under conditions of a colossal catastrophe. There is no one event, crisis, or meltdown to provide a convenient throughline. There is only an area, vast enough to be its own region, that hosted the most powerful explosions on Earth and where groups of people have learned to live with and embrace the past. It tells the story of Koian and of the fragile existence of the extended families and kin networks of stockbreeders who make a nuclear border zone their home. It's neither a heroic account of survival in extreme hardship nor a shocking tale of the decades of abuse at the hands of medical or military institutions (though both are true). Rather, what follows is an explanation of an exceptionally independent and original way of life that Koian residents have conceived for their daily existence – how they make a living, how they relate to the world outside, and why they chose to stay in contaminated lands. This is a story about what I call an *atomic collective*,[11] where mutual aid combined with fatalistic comradery enables the residents of Koian to shoulder medical, social, and economic practices that stigmatize them and turn that neglect into a virtue.

When I started my graduate studies in anthropology at the University of Colorado, Boulder, I certainly wasn't planning to spend the better part of my thirties in a dusty and isolated village near an abandoned nuclear test site far away from anywhere. Like most people, I had never even heard of the Semipalatinsk Test Site. When I first went to Kazakhstan in the summer of 2007, I was researching Polish diaspora communities – the children and grandchildren of people who were forcibly transferred by the Soviets from Poland's multi-ethnic eastern borderlands annexed during World War II by the paranoid and xenophobic Joseph Stalin. He mobilized thousands of his apparatchiks to ship "enemies of the state" in train cattle cars bound for the depths of Russia. My family was part of that group and was exiled to northern Kazakhstan on one Friday morning in 1939 from our home in the Grodno region (today part of Belarus). But unlike many of those who starved and froze to death, most of my relatives were lucky enough to survive and returned to Poland at the conclusion of the war, even while others were forbidden to leave. Today there are some fifty thousand self-identified Poles living in Kazakhstan. I wanted to understand why they retain a sense of ethnic identity despite decades of pressure to assimilate.

On this trip, a chance encounter changed the direction of my research. I met Semyon – Olek's boss. A passionate environmental activist and founder of one of the first and probably most successful organizations working to clean up hazardous waste in Kazakhstan, he was the first person to tell me about the Polygon. Ukrainian by birth and a radio-ecologist by training, he moved to Kazakhstan in the early 1990s. As one of the first liquidators sent to help clean up the Chornobyl (Chernobyl) nuclear accident in Ukraine, he was concerned about the health of people living on and near the Polygon. "It's the only place on Earth where people live next to craters produced by underground nuclear blasts, travel freely through some of the most radioactive areas on the planet, and work in mines in the territory," I vividly remember him saying. "But no one cares. It [the Polygon] is now 'open for business' since it was closed for testing." His organization has tried to force Kazakhstan's officials to move some of the villagers away from the test site and secure the most radioactive areas. Their efforts were met with resistance from state officials who didn't seem to care and communities that didn't want to move. So Semyon did what scientists do when there's nothing else that can be done – he printed radiation safety pamphlets with cartoon characters warning of danger.

I was puzzled by the rather jarring reality that people can and do live in a region where nuclear testing occurred. How was this even possible? Why do people stay? Aren't they worried about radiation? The chance meeting with Semyon and my "discovery" of the Polygon coincided with something more immediate in my life – how the radiation released during the Chornobyl (Chernobyl) catastrophe was affecting the health of the people closest to me. While my first memories of the accident are vague, I clearly remember the stomach-turning iodine drink my mother handed to me and the foul taste it left in my mouth.

I can also vividly recall everyone gathering outside for the celebratory May 1 International Workers' Day parade a mere five days after the accident. After emigrating to the United States in the late 1980s, my mother and grandmother discovered thyroid tumours, while my aunt's malignant renal carcinoma took her kidney. In 2007 my sister was diagnosed with cancer and eventually had her thyroid surgically removed. I couldn't help but be deeply puzzled by people living on the Polygon who seemingly were deliberately putting themselves in harm's way by refusing to leave when my family was convinced they were suffering from the after effects of radiation exposure that came from hundreds of kilometres away.

When I returned to Kazakhstan at the end of August 2010 to start my fieldwork, I didn't even know Koian existed. It's not listed on any available area maps and doesn't even show up on Google. Scientific peer-reviewed articles rarely (if ever) mention Koian, and the geneticists, epidemiologists, oncologists, and environmental activists who do work on the Polygon primarily focus on the larger settlements and villages studied by their Soviet-era predecessors. I had an ambitious project in mind: one year of fieldwork divided equally between three different villages on the border of the test site, followed by work with Semyon's organization and interviews with any activists, government officials, doctors, epidemiologists, and other local scientists willing to talk to me. The previous two years I had read as much as I could about Central Asia, Kazakhstan, and the Soviet Union. I learned about Hiroshima, Nagasaki, the Marshall Islands, French Polynesia, Nevada, the four corners region of the western United States, and other key places where downwind communities bore the brunt of radioactive fallout. I read about weapons laboratories and production facilities, uranium mining industries, nuclear waste sites, and places where major accidents also left lasting radioactive fallout. My adviser, as well as my American nuclear physicist and epidemiologist colleagues, encouraged me to learn how to use a Geiger counter and instructed me on how to best protect myself against radiation – what to eat, what to avoid, and how to put on a hazmat suit correctly. I even took a hazardous materials training class designed for those handling radioactive materials. I thought I was prepared.

But Semyon just roared with laughter when I arrived and presented my research plan to him. With decades of experience working in the region, he knew how to safely navigate the radioactive territory but more so what living in the region entailed. He pointed out that my plan hadn't reckoned dealing with the harsh continental climate, where temperatures often dip well below thirty degrees Fahrenheit (more than minus thirty degrees Celsius) in winter. I was also ignorant of the fact that many of the roads I had planned on travelling and carefully high-lighted on my map either no longer existed or are completely impassi-ble for much of the year and that there was no public transportation to get me where I wanted to be.

Insisting that I reconsider the structure of my project, Semyon sug-gested I limit my focus to the small village of Koian, because "it's a place ignored by everyone else, even though there's much to learn from the people who live so close to ground zero." Koian was also where he had completed his last project, and he knew the people there and could vouch for me. He even said his organization could probably find me if "something goes wrong." And so once again I pivoted and began draft-ing a new research plan.

Adjusting my research meant that most of September 2010 I spent pre-paring for departure. Semyon's organization and I pooled our money so I could buy a six-year-old blue diesel Mitsubishi Delica van with non-functional four-wheel drive (more perilous was the fact that it had a right-side steering wheel). Although the car belonged to the organiza-tion, it was mine for the duration of my stay, so long as I registered and insured it. After gathering various stamps in countless offices to com-plete the endless paperwork, I began to think of government officials as trained in psychological abuse. I gained a first-hand appreciation for what Koianers must go through to get anything done and came to appreciate their name for bureaucracy: *durakratiia*, or idiocracy (a pun on the Russian *byurokratiia*).

At the end of September, I set out for Koian with the car packed full of supplies – extra gas canisters, candles, shovels, ropes, spare tires, water, felt and rubber boots, masks, gloves, medical emergency kit, non-perishable food items, and countless other things I hadn't even consid-ered like a diesel fuel blowtorch (which I would soon learn how to use to heat the Delica's engine oil in winter when the car wouldn't start). What quickly became apparent is that the further away one is from the city, the worse conditions get. Roads are washed out, signs are either missing or incorrect, and gas stations become less and less frequent until they disappear entirely. After five hours, the asphalt road ends abruptly, becoming the much-loathed "grader" that decades ago was regularly maintained. Now it's eroded and potholed, the deep open gaps grabbing at the tires. Dust is everywhere, and my whole body vibrates and jostles the two hours it takes to traverse the thirty-mile (nearly fifty-kilometre) stretch until this road ends too at a dusty settlement of about three hundred people called Oktiabr'. After that, it's only the open steppe and an hour's worth of makeshift paths to Koian. Thankfully, Semyon has arranged for the mayor of Oktiabr' to meet me and lead the way from there. The mayor doubles as an excellent mechanic, teaching me how to change the first of what were more than twenty flat tires I would have to repair during my first year of fieldwork. In time, I would learn that in these parts it's necessary to become self-sufficient, and what looks like junk and scrap – like a three-hundred-pound concrete block or some rusty metal wire – could soon be put to good use weighing down the back of the Delica for extra traction and fastening the hatch so it wouldn't fly open.

The first time I saw Koian, it was like something out of an American Western. As if transported through time to 1870, horses stood on a hill against a backdrop of a perfectly still lake that looked like a silver disk made of salt. This was Kazakhstan's hill country, composed of craggy outcroppings that locals say look like an old man's wrinkled face after a poor night's sleep. Two old cemeteries and the concrete frames of large half-cylinders came into view as I approached the village – the skeletons of silos slowly being consumed by the grasses. In Koian, I was greeted by Tursynbek and his wife, Altynai, who were both in their mid-fifties. They soon became my adopted parents, and their guidance was indispensable to not only my work but for simply surviving in Koian. They not only fed me but taught me how to prepare the bathhouse, start a stove fire, limewash the walls of my one-room apartment, and recognize animals in the dark by the shine in their eyes.

My new home was a separate apartment attached to their main house. It consisted of four rooms, though only one was actually habitable. That room had everything I would need to make it through winter: a woodburning stove, a rusted bed frame, and a shelf. Most of the windows were either cracked or missing glass altogether, while the floorboards were so widely spaced that they let the field mice in (a problem I solved by getting a cat). There was no electricity until Tursynbek and his relatives ran a cable to power a single light bulb inside.

I would soon get to know all fifty residents of this windswept village and many more in Oktiabr' and other settlements. Like everyone else, my time was spent preparing food, washing clothes, keeping the house free of soot and mice, collecting cow dung or coal for fuel, fetching water, driving to the store, stockpiling supplies, pulling out vehicles sunk to the doors in mud, searching for missing livestock, and going to weddings, birthday parties, and funerals.

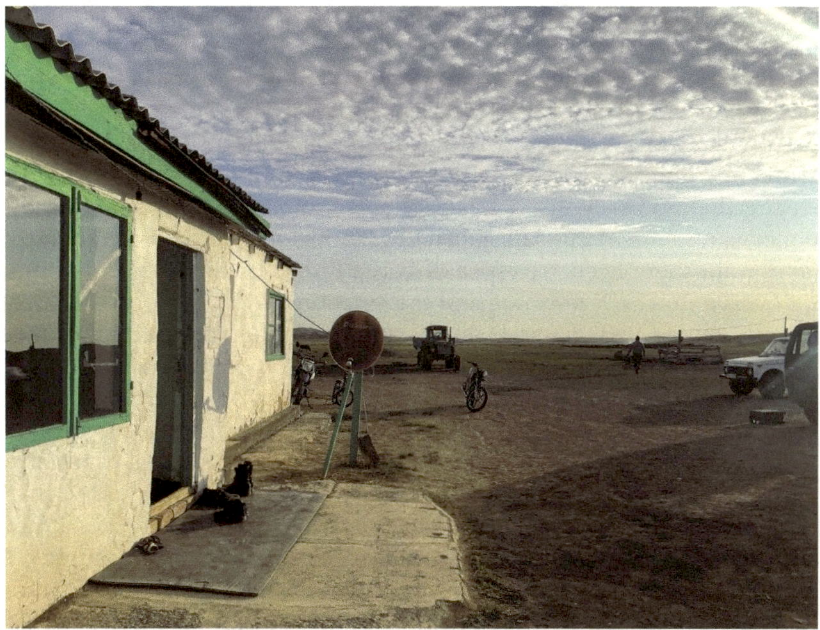

Figure I.3. *Last House on the Edge of the Polygon*. View from my home in Koian. The Polygon territory is visible on the distant horizon, several kilometres away.

This was my home from September 2010 to August 2011 and almost every subsequent summer for month-long follow-up visits until the COVID-19 pandemic upended my plans to visit in 2020.

Conducting an ethnography in such conditions meant certain choices were out of my hands. For example, I was a full-fledged member of the community during my time there and therefore engaged in "participant observation."[12] The choice of this approach not only was foisted upon me based on my circumstances but also was apt given my interest in the everyday experience of survival in "remote places" like Koian, often deemed peripheral to the study of nuclear politics.[13] Ethnography was also a good fit in light of its commitment to multi-vocality. In speaking and living among the residents of Koian, I sought a window that would allow me to see the radioactive afterlife of the Cold War through local accounts of everyday experiences. I wanted to understand how broader conceptual debates about the Cold War, risk, and competing scientific discourses about human and environmental effects of radiation exposure manifested in the lived experiences of actual people.

How the villagers of Koian navigate the aftermaths of the Cold War arms race that played out in their backyard is a sensitive topic.[14] To ensure their privacy and protect people from possible retaliation by police, government officials, journalists, mine operators, or neighbours (and grant them licence to speak freely), I have invented pseudonyms for everyone who lives there and the surrounding villages, even when people wanted to be named. Koian[15] itself is a real place but not its real name. At the same time, it's extremely difficult to anonymize a small village like Koian. For that reason, I have invented several individuals entirely by combining the biographies of two real people to protect their privacy at their request. All other places and names, especially those of public figures, remain unchanged.[16]

Although I began my time in Koian as a researcher with broad theoretical questions about health, radioactivity, and political economy, I soon learned that these questions took on a markedly different character in context. I discovered answers to these questions lay in how local mayors control the electricity for remote villages through favours and allegiance; how grassfires commonly sweep across the nuclear test site and send car loads of stock breeders with jugs of water and sheepskins to protect their fields; and how the "people of the Polygon" are shunned in cities, are abused in hospitals, and take jobs in mines where they are not permitted to measure radiation levels. Keen to create as three-dimensional a picture of Koian as I could, I sought out as many interview subjects as possible, and eventually conducted over one hundred in-depth semi-structured and informal interviews primarily in Russian with residents, physicians, environmental activists and government officials, as well as nuclear physicists, radioecologists, epidemiologists and other scientists working on nuclear-related issues. Although focused on Koian, I didn't limit my search for answers to just the village and travelled to multiple locations – and even through the Polygon – searching out answers to the questions I found myself asking.

I also found myself spending long hours in archives, poring over all manner of documents in search of data I could use. Because I was investigating how political, economic, social, and scientific forces animated life on the Polygon, there was a wealth of data to consider: demographic, statistical and policy documents generated by the Kazakh state, the Russian Federation, international organizations such as the International Atomic Energy Agency, the World Health Organization, and the Organisation for Economic Co-operation and Development, as well as US government agencies working on the prevention of the spread of nuclear weapons. My research also benefited from archival data that I gathered at the Hoover Institution Library and Archives, State Archive of Karaganda, National Archive in Astana, and the Central State Archive of the Republic of Kazakhstan in Almaty, as well as smaller archives in other cities and those held at several museums in the region.

What I learned reading those documents sent me back into the field to ask additional questions. For example, my analysis of state strategy in Kazakhstan for dealing with residual radioactivity draws on documentary analysis from multiple archives cross-referenced against interviews with government officials in charge of environmental protection and economic development, as well as city and village mayors. My interest in acute and low-dose radiation exposure not only led me into the medical literature on the topic but also sent me on trips across the country to Karaganda, Astana, Almaty, and Semey interviewing physicians and scientists specializing in illnesses related to radioactive exposure. And to experience firsthand what it was like to work at a Kazakhstan-based environmental organization devoted to improving the lives of Koianers, I spent four months as a participant observer with them in Karaganda, where I read their internal and published documents, attended meetings, and collaborated on a variety of projects related to environmental issues stemming from nuclear testing.

Atomic Collective is a historical, theoretical, and ethnographic study of the sociocultural consequences of the Soviet atomic bomb project in Kazakhstan told by those most affected yet least understood. My work is a close-up of life in a nuclear zone – what the Indigenous Kazakh residents refer to as both the "good life" and a challenging one. This book asks two main questions: what compels people to stay in a region where nuclear testing occurred, and by what means do they do it?

From this overarching question, *Atomic Collective* offers an intimate look at the links between Cold War nuclear weapons testing and the political, economic, and social worlds that have emerged in the post–Soviet era. It shows the exceptionally independent and original way of life that extended families and kin networks of stockbreeders in Koian have reconceived for their daily existence – how they make a living, how they relate to the world outside, and how they understand their health. Rather than seeing chronic illness as a means to access state resources, as has happened in other post-Soviet contexts (most notably Chornobyl/Chernobyl)[17] and in other contexts where such weapons were tested,[18] what distinguishes the residents of the Polygon is how they have "embraced" radiation and its purported effects over time as a sign of their own genetic resilience.[19] The research behind *Atomic Collective* opens a larger vantage point to show that there is no uniform way that victimhood or the biological effects of radioactive pollution are understood (even including among scientists) and thus no consensus regarding what are safe and unsafe places to live. As a result, Indigenous Kazakh residents have been left during the post-Soviet period to navigate the economic austerity, cultural marginalization, and environmentally linked health anxieties of where they live on their own. More than a century of shifting political structures and ideologies have indelibly left their mark.[20]

Atomic Collective approaches nuclear testing and its socio-cultural legacies historically. The timeline stretches from the 1949 start of the Soviet program in Kazakhstan up through the present. The narrative arc that emerges from the life history of residents spans several key aspects of the post-Soviet period, including tensions over environmental history, the legacies of state secrecy, neoliberal market transitions, and scientific uncertainty about the health effects of low-dose and chronic radiation exposure. It offers a deep look at how the neoliberal and scientific domains in Kazakhstan have themselves mutated after the fall of the Soviet Union as a result of political and economic restructuring, the absence of policy, and outright denial of the truth. Bringing these threads together unearths a social structure born out of the Soviet collapse, in which Kazakhstan's inability to deal with billions of tons of inherited toxic waste coupled with the economic opportunities presented across a variety of industrial sectors have created the conditions for an inhabited but unregulated radioactive landscape.

Informed by my extensive research, I selected a conceptual framework and theoretical orientation for thinking about my findings that was primarily indebted to political and economic perspectives in cultural anthropology and critical medical anthropology. For obvious reasons, my research in Koian both recognizes and foregrounds marginalized communities within broader socio-economic dynamics.[21] My goal in looking at Koian is to contribute to and engage public anthropology[22] in its commitment to reframing debates – in my case to reframing questions such as the relationship among economics, politics, and health in the context of "nuclearity."[23]

This book highlights how nuclearity (the shifting quality of something to be nuclear) in Kazakhstan shapes debates about nuclear victimhood and the health impacts of radiation exposure. It also examines the intricate interplay between economics, politics, and health during the transformation from a socialist to a neoliberal order within the Soviet legacy, and at the peripheries of nuclear history and imperialism.[24] Anthropologists studying communities affected by nuclear fallout often grapple with understanding how people navigate their circumstances. Most look for collective actions or some form of organized resistance, hoping for people to fight for what is right and challenge established authority.[25] For instance, the Marshall Islanders have made some headway in seeking justice after nuclear testing took place on their homeland.[26] However, these efforts often encounter obstacles, and occasionally researchers confront a sense of fatalism or collective inaction. In many cases, people would rather have opportunities in the places they live rather than give up their home for "clean" environments. For example, the lead communities in Argentina documented by sociologist Javier Auyero and anthropologist Debora Swistun,[27] and anthropologist Daniel Renfrew's[28] examination of lead communities in Uruguay have similarities. In the context of Chornobyl (Chernobyl), there is also an assumption that disenfranchised populations, who lack power, experience post-Soviet "fatalism," appearing too passive when faced with challenges, leading to a development of a maladaptive "sick society" characterized by corruption, injustice, or moral decay.[29]

But the broader story of Kazakhstan's social and cultural nuclear legacies also offers a unique window into post-socialist[30] societies once colonized by the Soviet Union. By focusing on the anthropology of local and global toxic environmental catastrophes and how these disproportionately affected and (re)produced the marginalized citizens of Koian, what I have written here also contributes to a wide array of literatures, including those that look at risk and uncertainty, environmental crisis, ruination as a lived experience, resource exploitation, and health effects across social sciences.[31] Because Koian sits at the intersection of environmental, political, and economic crises, researching it has led me into the realm of nuclear humanities, where the landscapes of late capitalism polluted with "invisible harms"[32] fall within the context of scientific uncertainty to shape health risks in the nuclear age.[33]

My fieldwork touches on politics in a variety of ways. As the first ethnography to examine communities in Kazakhstan living in and around the Polygon and the ways they confront and make sense of their lives, it illustrates the effects of unrestrained neoliberalism and uncertain science on political decision making. Just under the surface of Koianers' day-to-day existence are post-Soviet regulatory regimes and "scientific expertise" masquerading as fact – shaping both the social practices and subjectivities of individuals living in and around the Polygon.[34] While past studies of the Polygon address issues of "risk perceptions" and memory work[35] as well as state and local strategies of knowing and not knowing the site,[36] this book squarely addresses the gap in the literature as it pertains to the areas of health, science, and invisible environmental toxicity in Central Asia.[37] The book adds to the ongoing debates on the role of regime change and "transition" politics in shaping civil society in post-Soviet states.[38] It also contributes to debates about the relationship between politics and economics, exploring how power and resources are distributed and controlled and how people deal with crises.[39]

Although environmental crisis plays an important role in the politics of other Central Asian republics and former Soviet states, the situation is particularly acute in Kazakhstan, where rural populations experience a higher burden stemming from the simultaneous nuclear and economic legacies of the Soviet era. The effects are vividly felt in and around Koian, and accordingly *Atomic Collective* speaks directly to the scholarship on globalization and health by shifting the lens from broad effects like employment insecurity and devaluation as reasons for high morbidity to examine at the ground level how economic transformations disproportionally affect contaminated rural communities.[40] I examine how scientific practice mutates as it encounters different social, political, and economic domains so as to legitimate the view that the former nuclear test site is "clean" and claims of ill health are morphed more into questions about individual mental stability than exposure to residual radioactivity itself.

Atomic Collective provides a detailed case study of the nuclear legacies of the Soviet atomic bomb program, from ruination as a lived experience to colonial militarization.[41] But Kazakhstan in particular offers a unique vantage point on elements of nuclear politics absent in contexts like the United States – namely the role of state and corporate actors in co-producing radioactive living spaces and the people who have come to accept it. Given that Kazakhstan suffered the loss of half its population and was turned into a hub of labour camps and exile during the Stalinist era, the influence of Soviet state power on the subjectivity and daily life of Koianers cannot be overstated. Yet a straightforward narrative of the Sovietization of Kazakhstan is misleading at best.[42] After all, if Soviet leaders were truly able to shape the subjectivity of Kazakhs, why did they resort to such excessive violence? Good subjects should willingly comply with authority without the need for coercion, believing that they are acting of their own accord. In fact, a closer look at the Soviet and post–Soviet era in places like Koian reveals a curious mix of state interest and neglect – a combination of intense investment in certain aspects of life in remote settlements paired with residents being largely left to their own devices. When Soviet nuclear testing began, Koian was a collective farm without electricity, glass windows, proper housing, or trade. Between the mid-1950s and 1989, the state made major contextual changes related to agriculture extension, markets, and military technologies – providing villagers with money, coal, and food in exchange for enduring bombs and serving as living medical experiments. But with the cessation of testing, the state left the villagers to fend for themselves – what the philosopher Giorgio Agamben[43] refers to as a "naked life," progressively stripped of protection and political rights. This experience is what my narrative captures; namely, the exceptional self-sufficiency and originality with which Koian residents go about their existence.

The gradual erosion of basic human necessities leads to the striking realization that the people of Koian have given up on making any demands for their rights or services as citizens. They do not request roads, the restoration of schools, emergency services, or medicine and have no expectations of access to uncontaminated food and clean land. They do not anticipate a healthy life for themselves or their children. But rather than wallow in victimhood, seek justice, or pursue empowerment through cultural revival (as in the case of the Marshall Islanders),[44] what emerges is a remarkable story of resilience in the face of such catastrophic events in a place of constant crisis. Their passivity seems so profound as to announce a complete social and psychological collapse, leading outsiders to perceive them as existing in a state of miserable limbo. And yet a closer look reveals them as seemingly defying Agamben's description of "goners" in *Homo Sacer*. Koianers see what looks like indifference to outsiders as toughness and strength.

Atomic Collective expands on Agamben's ideas by delving into the reasoning and mindset of Koian residents, giving them greater depth and humanity than the shades of naked life that Agamben discusses and projects into the twenty-first century. Although the ability of the Polygon communities to confront and understand their past, present, and future is constrained by their access to information as a result of Soviet-era secrecy and limited power in decision-making processes,[45] the book reveals a people who nevertheless remain defiant in their desire and ability to eke out an existence on the margins of the Polygon. If there was a core of Koianers' existence that I was able to identify, in it would lie a collective refusal not only to conform or participate in established power structures[46] but to refuse to feel stigmatized and excluded. Koianers consistently push back against and challenge social, political, and economic structures, often using subtle forms of agency that give shape to their sense of autonomy. Central to their collective repudiation is a shared awareness of myriad outside pressures and influences that are threatening to their way of life and the vision of a cultural identity born in the midst of a chaotic landscape marked by precarity. Koianers constantly negotiate boundaries and limitations and despite it all, the persistence of the village illuminates the ability of marginalized communities to snub definitions made by others, and actively nurture their own social and cultural contexts.

Atomic Collective consists of four chapters and a conclusion. In Chapter 1, "'The Forbidden Zone': Atomic Bombs and the Good Life," I delve into the rich history of Koian through the eyes of its residents. The chapter blends locally significant narratives with archival evidence to give a comprehensive view of the region's history, including Koian's formerly nomadic life, Russia's colonial expansion, and Soviet nuclear testing and agricultural development. This context-driven perspective offers a deeper understanding of the diverse ways in which people narrate their past and sets the stage for the investigations that follow.

Chapter 2, "'Clean Air Is Our Death': Debates about Genetic Mutation" probes deeper into understanding why people are not afraid of radiation and their decision to remain close to the test site. The farmland and bodies of Koianers were contaminated by Soviet nuclear testing, but they have transformed this fact into a virtue by justifying their continued exposure to radiation as essential for their survival. Koianers acknowledge that this exposure has come at a high cost to their health and well-being, but they still embrace it. This chapter is a critical examination of the role of scientific debates on low-dose radiation and the interplay among these debates, the inhabited radioactive landscape, and how this shapes the residents' perception of their own biology and subjectivity. The concept of "radiophobia" is also explored, with an examination of how social, cultural, and historical factors have shaped its deployment on the Polygon. The chapter aims to provide a comprehensive understanding of the complexities of living in scientific uncertainty and an inhabited radioactive landscape.

Chapter 3, "'Sami Po Sebe': Economy on the Periphery," sheds light on the unique economic challenges faced by Polygon communities by focusing on the determination of Koianers, who despite facing economic difficulties after the collapse of the Soviet command economy, refuse to give up their collective farm. The institution that their grandparents were forced to join and that used to provide them with what they remember was a decent wage, has quite literally been stolen out from under them by former administrators. But Koianers have transformed their unemployment into an opportunity by exploiting the free market potential of the Polygon, despite the evident hazards involved. This chapter examines how the villagers have adapted to the post-Soviet agro-nuclear landscape by establishing informal economies and using social networks, both of which play an important role in ameliorating a lack of state commitment to the region, with the curious result of the village becoming a relatively stable economic unit and a linchpin in a broader strategy of upward mobility for family members who move to cities.

In Chapter 4, "'They Think We Are Stupid': Reinventing Kazakh Tradition," I examine how Koianers are perceived outside the village and navigate symbolic violence directed against them. During Imperial Russia's rule, nomads were confined to summer and winter pastures, and later Soviet regulations on passports resulted in a perpetual village confinement, making it difficult for individuals to relocate to urban areas without official approval (often linked to formal education and demonstrated loyalty to the Soviet Union). Despite their ancestors' nomadic lifestyle, Koianers have embraced their enforced settlement in one village and have redefined ancestral duty as staying rather than migrating. This chapter delves into how the treatment by the scientific and medical communities has only reinforced the villagers' determination to remain in the village and make a virtue out of their enforced settlement. I show how their individual and collective actions to refuse the legitimacy of the authorities and outsiders allowed Koianers to simultaneously exist outside post-Soviet hierarchical social relations and not to be defined by others.

In the Conclusion, "The Atomic Present," I return to the themes of the book, pushing beyond the boundaries of meta-narratives about "victimhood" and environmental crisis by pointing to the broader implications of life in radioactive ruins, reflecting on the way Koianers have come to see their lives in light of extreme hardship and tragedy. Although Koianers appear to dwell in what outsiders see as an abject limbo, I argue that they have transformed their hardships into strengths and the vices they have been subjected to into remarkable virtues.

1 "The Forbidden Zone": Atomic Bombs and the Good Life

The tradition of the oppressed teaches us that the "state of emergency" in which we live is not the exception but the rule.

– Walter Benjamin, On the Concept of History

Introduction

Before my arrival in Koian in 2010, I had only a partial idea of what the Soviet Union's primary nuclear test site looked like. A few photographs, a couple of documentary films, some news reports and government publications, and the opinions of my urban interlocutors in Kazakhstan produced in me a medley of post-apocalyptic images. But I also had something concrete that helped me see the invisible – the first publicly available map of the Polygon that depicted the extent of radioactive pollution in the region.

Since Semyon and his environmental organization were helping me settle in Koian, I was asked to provide copies to villagers as part of an education campaign promoting radiation safety. With its dark-red border demarcating the extent of the test site, it showed Koian and many other villages dotting the edge. Circled in green indicating that the villages are safe to inhabit, some are located just a few kilometres from the still dangerous *slied* (trace) left by an atomic bomb that exploded more than six decades earlier on September 24, 1951. The radioactive footprint was denoted in a lighter shade of red and stretched from ground zero in the north part of the site southward for about seventy miles (about 130 kilometres).

But even that map wasn't free from imaginative projection. In small print at the bottom of the map was the following message:

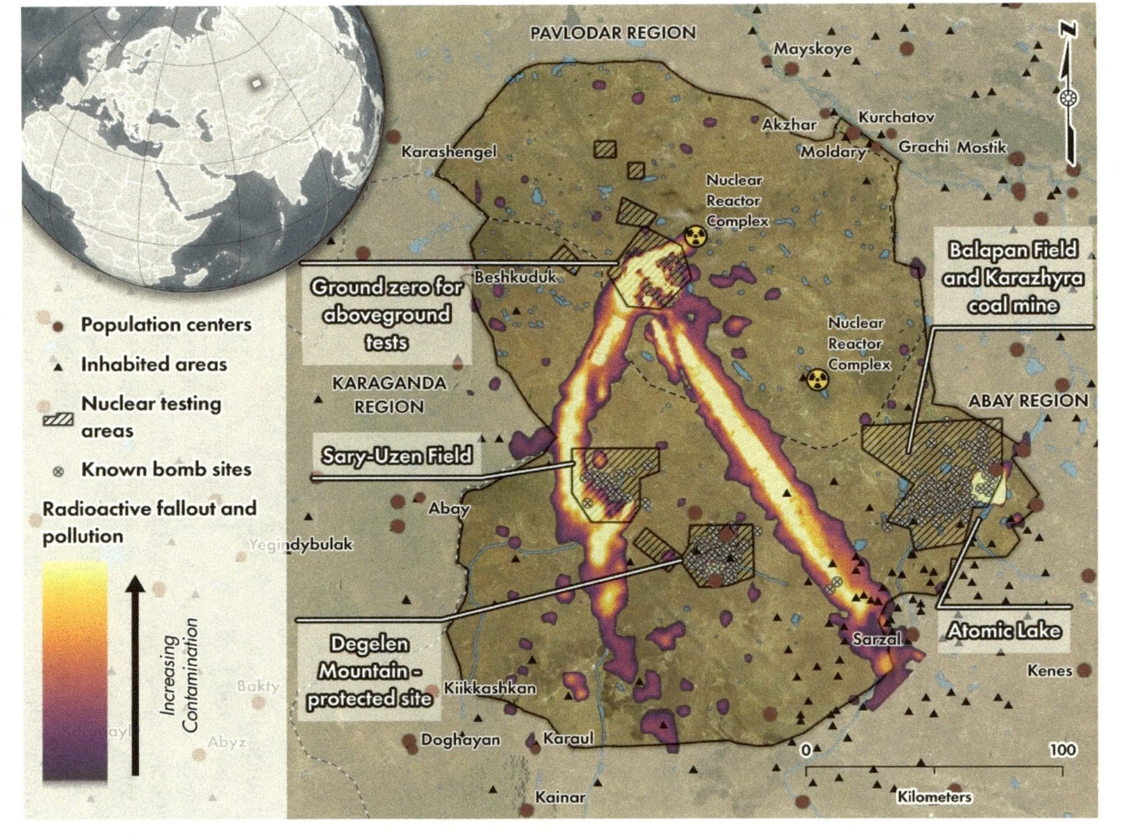

Map 2. Polygon

This map has been prepared and published with the financial support
of the OSCE Centre in Almaty. The OSCE Centre in Almaty shall in no
circumstances be responsible for the accuracy and authenticity of the information and data it contains. The boundaries and names on this map,
which originate from a variety of open-source material, do not imply in
any form or fashion an official endorsement or acceptance by the Organisation for Security and Co-operation in Europe (OSCE).

As I came to learn later, the areas of radiation pollution noted on the
map are quite incomplete and even grossly inaccurate at points, and the
map had an initial print run of only five hundred copies. This is not for
lack of effort on OSCE's part: some of the radiation data remain classified, and the National Nuclear Center of the Republic of Kazakhstan rejected their first map, claiming that not all radioactive areas have been
studied properly. As a result, only radioactive traces from two above-
ground explosions from the test site were represented and two resulting areas of high radioactive contamination. First-hand experience also
revealed that the Polygon boundaries on the map don't physically exist
in any visible sense and that many settlements on the map have been
abandoned, while others are not shown at all. The five roads depicted
converging on Koian were also an illusion unless one considers various
dirt paths of the open steppe as candidates. Although the map was far
from perfect, it was also the only one available to the public and the
only one the environmental organization was allowed to print. That
told me two key things right at the start of my investigation that have
held true ever since: there is a lack of reliable information about the
former nuclear test site, and the only way to fill in those gaps would
be through soliciting local knowledge of the landscape. But the map I
wound up discovering over the course of my inquiries created something completely different from a flat two-dimensional representation
of a radioactive site.

As instructed by Semyon, I brought a poster tube full of these maps
to Koian. The one I hung on the wall of my room quickly became a vibrant conversation piece that ironically would have nothing to do with
the atomic testing represented on the map. On countless occasions, I
learned about everything that was not present: nearby mountains,
lakes, rivers, fishing areas, Polygon swimming holes, villages, mining
operations, the best pasturelands, ancestral sites, and former collective farm areas, and which routes to take while travelling to each of
these places. I also heard stories of everything villagers believed was a
state secret: airports, army training grounds, nuclear craters, and mining ventures operating in the region. I quickly came to realize that for

villagers the map was a staging ground for demonstrating wide-ranging local knowledge about the area – a contest between who is a *mestnyi* (a local) and who is a *ne mestnyi* (not local) – but that rarely touched on the topic of Soviet-era nuclear testing. In fact, during most of my fieldwork, I had to prompt conversations about nuclear testing and its effects on local Koian residents. Once the conversation was initiated, most people were eager to share with me their life stories of survival and betrayal, but much to my surprise, residents also told stories of a good life on the Polygon that they highlighted in the kaleidoscopic meanings attached to places.[1]

Before the Bombs

Koian has a pre-Soviet and even a pre-Russian history that can be seen in the area's centuries-old rocky grave mounds and boulders with faded pictographs that conceivably date back a thousand years or more. On my excursions into the steppe with Tursynbek, I've seen little paintings of a Bactrian camel, a horse with a rider, and a bunch of mountain goats trailed by a dog or maybe a wolf.

Traditionally, Kazakhs were nomads grouped in *auls* (small clan units), a term still used to refer to small Kazakh settlements like Koian, consisting of several families. They migrated with their animals along annual routes to pasture, paying respects to ancestors buried along the way. Many locals can trace their ancestry in the area back seven generations and most are kin belonging to clans of the Middle Horde, famous for its intellectuals, philosophers, and artists.[2] Kazakh kinship is based on patrilineal descent, clan exogamy, and patrilocal residence, meaning that Koianers trace their ancestry through the male line, while women marry outside their clan group and settle with their husband's family.[3] Although extremely isolated groups remained outside the reach of the Russian Empire's economic development and colonizing "civilizing" missions that began in the mid-eighteenth century, Tsarist settlement practices nevertheless ultimately restricted nomads to just their summer and winter pastures.[4] Koian became a settlement by the virtue of the fact that nomads were no longer free to migrate long distances and had to stake out some ground or lose it. Elders claimed that once Koian's clans settled, the aul became a *beket* – a horse-swapping station between postal points during the Tsarist period. Their pastoral life today is seen by them as a return to some degree to the life their nomadic ancestors lived.[5]

The October Revolution of 1917 in Russia had overthrown the Tsar and had a profound impact on Central Asia. The new Bolshevik-led leadership sought to radically reconstruct an entire society anew. When the Bolsheviks "liberated" Kazakhstan from Tsarist oppression in 1920, they added it to a growing list of territories slated for radical development along socialist lines.[6] Following Marxist-Leninist dictum, the communists viewed Kazakhstan as the most backward of all regions in the Union, one inhabited by "prehistoric" shepherds and nomads stuck somewhere between primitive communism and slavery.[7] In the eyes of the 1920s Soviet leadership, nomadism was the most exploitative and thus lowest form of social and economic organization, one in need of complete eradication if the region and its people were to become properly Soviet modern.[8] Although the nomadic lifestyle was never fully eradicated in Kazakhstan by the Bolsheviks and was sometimes even implicitly supported by the state, the goal was to ultimately reconstitute Kazakhstan as an exemplary Soviet Socialist Republic and showcase the eventual achievement of modernity through education – proof that even the most "primitive" peoples of the world can be compelled to evolve.[9] Koian and its people were therefore assimilated into the vast Soviet modernizing project, experiencing firsthand the paradigmatic changes and challenges of socialist planning.

As told by those who experienced the rapid transformation first-hand as very young children or having heard about it from their parents, the violent attack on the Kazakh way of life began shortly after 1928.[10] The Soviet leader Joseph Stalin introduced repressive measures designed to rapidly industrialize the Soviet Union. These included an all-out forced collectivization of peasant agriculture, expropriation and redistribution of grain and livestock, sedentarization of nomadic peoples, and deportation or murder of wealthy *bai* (rich herders) perceived as "enemies of the state."[11] The rapid pace of these transformations proved devastating. With livestock and grain confiscated, a famine killed nearly half of the Indigenous population – approximately 1.5 million ethnic Kazakhs, with the northern regions of Kazakhstan most strongly impacted.[12] There, three-quarters of the population either died or fled. In total, some 1.1 million Kazakhs fled to Russia, Kyrgyzstan, Mongolia, and Afghanistan.

Although most Koianers today were either born after the tragic famine years (1930–33) or were very young when it happened, I frequently heard stories about it over dinner, which people would say is eaten heartily today out of defiance of the Soviet regime and in remembrance of perished relatives. Tursynbek, who was born in Koian in the late 1950s, would tell me about the famine when I refused to eat more food. "It must have been 1932 or thereabouts. There was massive hunger here. We protested too! Collectivization was confiscation. But you don't want to eat? In Koian people ate each other," he would say, nodding sharply at my empty plate and the large communal bowl of food before us. Whether he was speaking metaphorically or whether cannibalism actually occurred during the famine years is unclear, and I didn't want to appear to be impolite by asking how Tursynbek's parents survived. With my radiation anxieties purged in lieu of hunger, I picked at the pieces of my favourite goat meat hidden beneath noodles piled high in the bowl and instead asked what happened to the animals. "They were confiscated. Then there was no food and whole villages were wiped out. People ate dogs, rats, even grass – everything they could get their hands on. Eventually, food ran out, so people had no choice but to eat other people, but we don't like to talk about that. Dead bodies were everywhere."

The effects of forced collectivization and sedentarization campaigns in Koian are vividly documented in archival sources.[13] In 1929 in the location of Koian, there were 6553 ethnic Kazakhs living in one of the six *raiony* (districts) that were subordinated to a larger administrative *okrug* (region), but by 1935 the population of the same region had fallen to 3863.[14] The animal numbers are even starker: in 1930 the entire region had 1,684,043 heads of livestock (including horses, sheep, goats, and even camels), but by the start of 1935, this number had been reduced to a measly 88,285, the animals either dying of hunger for lack of feed because of the collectivization of farming or were killed and eaten to avoid confiscation.[15]

By 1935, Koian and nearly 98.2 per cent of all settlements in the *okrug* belonged to a *kolkhoz*, a small collective farm cooperative.[16] Koian's kolkhoz consisted of at least eight separate villages or auls (from the name of the former migrating unit), each occupied by a number of extended families. The *kolkhozniki* (collective farm workers) in theory received a share of meat and dairy products according to the amount they worked and the number of people in their families. In reality, the new kolkhozy were a far cry from the gleaming reflections of Soviet planning in action; rather, their poor organization, coupled with a scarcity of resources, meant that people were mostly left to fend for themselves.

Burkut, in his eighties and Koian's oldest resident when I interviewed him in 2011, was six years old when Koian was collectivized. He still remembered those years vividly:

Originally, there were two kolkhozy here in Koian. Behind the hill there were two more and four more over that hill there, but we worked together. [After the famine] there was maybe a hundred people in total. Life was very hard because our herds were small – my father had one cow and

raised sheep for the kolkhoz. At the end of each year, the state requisi-
tioned sheep, and we were typically given one or two of the sick ones as
payment. We did whatever the administration told us to do. Otherwise,
we risked arrest. We still grazed our animals in the traditional way by
taking them out to pasture. There was never enough food. We had to steal
grain and hide it from the authorities. Until the early 1950s, we barely
survived. We lived in small houses built from adobe brick or sometimes
in yurts. The houses that are in Koian today were built much later. There
were no glass windows at the time – we used a thin mesh made from animal parts instead.[17]

Before Soviet atomic testing in 1949, Koian was a floundering kolkhoz
with no modern amenities like electricity, nor was it connected to any
larger trade networks (in part because like today there were no roads
to it). In his interview, Burkut revealed that he only learned about the
existence of money in the 1950s. For all intents and purposes, devel-
opmentally speaking, Koian was not that different from its Tsarist-era
incarnation. Historian Adeeb Khalid[18] observed that despite the nine-
teenth-century Russian and Chinese colonization of Central Asia leading to increased global connections in trade and ideas, early foreign
conquest was never capable of bringing about "radical cultural change"
in the region.[19] His point holds as well when discussing extremely rural
places like Koian in the early years of the Soviet era.

But the village history recounted to me in interviews describing the
time after the kolkhoz was transformed into a vast farm does note a turning point. In a kind of paradoxical trade-off – bombs for a good life – the
state began using villagers for war games and living radiation experiments, all in secret, and gave them money, coal, and hay in return.[20] The
sudden change in their circumstances was a product of two tandem projects of the Soviet period: nuclear testing and the Virgin Lands campaign.

Atomic Testing and the Virgin Lands Project

In 1947, the architects of the Soviet atomic bomb project began construction of their primary nuclear proving ground: the Semipalatinsk
Test Site named after the large city (today Semey) about eighty miles
(nearly 130 kilometres) directly east of the site. The verdant banks of
the Irtysh River, a little over sixty miles (about one hundred kilometres)
from Koian, were chosen as the "empty" and therefore "perfect" location for the command centre of this top-secret military installation.[21]
Known as Moscow-400, it was presented on publicly available maps as
the end of a railroad line and nothing more.[22] This administrative centre

that would later become Kurchatov (renamed in honour of the Soviet nuclear physicist who oversaw the Soviet bomb project) was a closed and secret city. Isolated from the outside world by strict controls on the mail and telephone, only those specially permitted could enter. People were even buried elsewhere. The extent of scientific and military activities remained a mystery except to the privileged consortium composed of Soviet administrators working on the bomb project. Yet despite its alleged secrecy, its existence and the forty-year period of nuclear testing that followed were well known to the local populations who worked on collective farms nearby.

For the next four decades, more than 450 above- and underground nuclear explosions at the Semipalatinsk Test Site research complex punctuated life in Koian and its nearby villages.[23] The frequency of the tests was remarkable – eight above-ground detonations alone during the month of October 1954.[24] Koian effectively became a secret military zone in 1947, and like Moscow-400 it too was erased from all publicly available maps. Because state secrets needed to be protected, the level of surveillance in the kolkhoz increased significantly. In short order, deep trenches and barbed wire fencing with mysterious signs announcing *Zona* (the Zone) appeared along Koian's test site boundary. Altynai, who worked on the farm, found the signs a curiosity. "We used to collect hay on the Polygon. I remember seeing signs that had zona (zone) written on them. We used to laugh about this. What sort of zone was this? *Zona otdykha* (a resort) perhaps? No one in the village had a clue."

Whereas before movement was restricted and policed by the kolkhoz supervisor, with Soviet passport regulations placing people under a perpetual village arrest in which moving to an urban area required official approval, after 1947 the military took an active role too.[25] Movement in the area was monitored, and only those working on collective farms were allowed to enter certain areas of the Polygon with prior military approval. I was told those who entered without proper authorization were promptly arrested.

While the rest of the Soviet society practised civil defence drills and learned how to protect themselves against a nuclear attack, people living in and around the Polygon knew nothing.[26] There were no bomb shelters, no gas masks, and no US-style "duck and cover" drills. "What they were doing on the Polygon, no one told us. Some of the soldiers wore gas masks, but we didn't know why," Burkut said.

Those who remember the tests told me that before each explosion, Soviet military troops would be dispatched to the region with safety instructions like the following: all stove fires were to be put out; all chimneys on all homes were to be covered; all water wells were to be sealed; all animals were to be corralled in one area; and all residents were to leave their homes until testing was complete. Zhanbolat, who was a teenager when he first saw a test, described it this way:

> Koian became a *zapreshchena zona* [forbidden zone] in 1946 and all sorts of [Soviet] soldiers came. This was the first time we saw soldiers – how were we supposed to know what a soldier looks like when we had never seen one? I was in the first grade. And then, I think, in 1954 atmospheric testing began and more soldiers started coming. Two or three lived here – they had their own food rations and generators. At the time in these lands, there was no electricity. The day of the explosion, soldiers stationed in Koian had to protect us so that nothing bad would happen. And we saw the bomb: oy, how the earth shook; and the brightness! Then a mushroom cloud appeared, followed by a loud noise. They only tested bombs when the wind blew away from the village for our own protection. It was all a secret. Then tests stopped in the atmosphere and went underground. They did those tests in two places. A huge crater appeared nearby, and we call it an atomic lake. I wasn't scared of the aboveground explosions, but I didn't like underground tests because those bombs were tested year-round and made a lot of noise.

Older residents like Zhanbolat remember feeling trembling under their feet like an earthquake and returning home to find things disturbed, with furniture out of place and objects having fallen from shelves. Yet for the residents of Koian, nuclear tests were overall a minor if unexplained interruption to the daily agricultural routine – mere inconveniences when people were asked to stop everything they were doing until after the testing was complete.

Starting in the mid-1950s, many people who lived in this manufactured, open-air laboratory were also (unbeknown to them) enrolled in clandestine human radiation research. Using the local parlance, the workers on state farms became the military-scientific establishment's "experimental rabbits." In the process, their health became a means of producing knowledge. There is no evidence that the Soviet authorities planned in advance to carry out protracted human experiments, but they nevertheless harvested data from the residents. The authorities secretly monitored thousands of people throughout the region for adverse signs of radiation exposure and, in 1957, established a secret clinic to lead this project.[27] In the nearby city of Semipalatinsk, medical doctors supervised by the Soviet Ministry of Health worked in a drab building under the pseudonym Anti-Brucellosis Dispensary No. 4 and reported their research directly to Moscow.[28] They pretended to treat

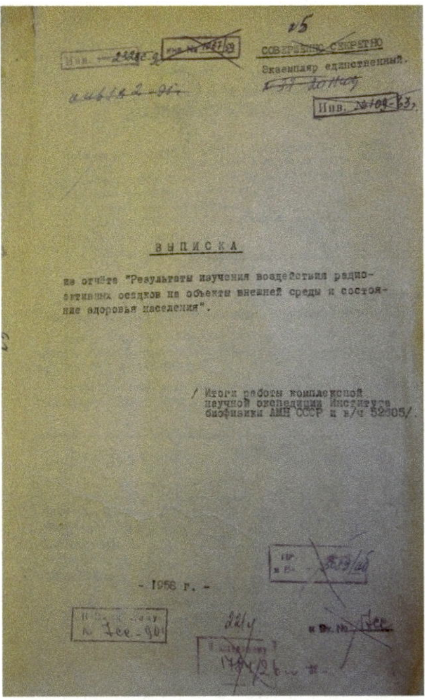

Figure 1.1. *Top Secret Report.* A 1958 report from an expedition led by the Institute of Biophysics working out of Dispensary No. 4, titled "The Results of Studying the Impact of Radioactive Fallout on Environmental Objects and the Health of the Population." In the upper-right-hand corner of the page, the text reads "TOP SECRET" and below, "Single copy," indicating it's the only existing print.

zoonotic diseases – those transmitted from animals to humans – but in fact assessed the impact of nuclear tests on public health, cataloged radiation-induced illnesses, and took note of death rates.[29]

Like the radiation coming from the landscape, the longitudinal and intergenerational data they collected on how exposure manifests itself in the human body were a state secret.[30] First-hand accounts from medical doctors I interviewed at local hospitals (and confirmed by a variety of archival and secondary sources I consulted) reported fainting, nosebleeds, diarrhoea, and/or hair loss – all tell-tale symptoms of acute radiation sickness.[31]

But residents were not permitted to speak of explosions nor any illness they suspected to be linked to them. Instead, individuals were

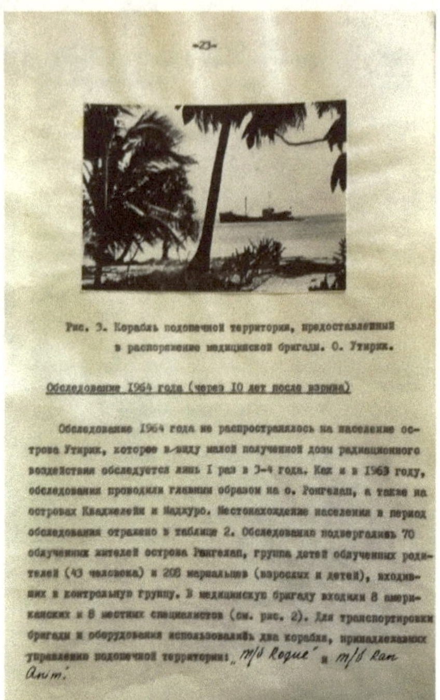

Рис. 3. Корабль подопечной территории, предоставленный
в распоряжение медицинской бригады. О. Утирик.

Обследование 1964 года (через 10 лет после взрыва)

Обследование 1964 года не распространялось на население острова Утирик, которое в виду малой полученной дозы радиационного воздействия обследуется лишь 1 раз в 3–4 года. Как и в 1963 году, обследования проводили главным образом на о. Ронгелап, а также на островах Кваджелейн и Маджуро. Местонахождение населения в период обследования отражено в таблице 2. Обследованию подвергались 70 облученных жителей острова Ронгелап, группа детей облученных родителей (43 человека) и 208 нормальных (взрослых и детей), входивших в контрольную группу. В медицинскую бригаду входили 8 американских и 8 местных специалистов (см. рис. 2). Для транспортировки бригады и оборудования использовались два корабля, принадлежащих управлению подопечной территории: „m/s Rogue" и m/s Ran Anim.

Figure 1.2. *Medical Survey of the Marshall Islands*. A 1965 translated report from English to Russian, released by the Brookhaven National Laboratory under contract with the United States Atomic Energy Commission, documenting research on the human impact of nuclear weapons testing at the Marshall Islands. The report is titled *Medical Survey of the People of Rongelap and Utirik Islands Nine and Ten Years after Exposure to Fallout Radiation (March 1963 and March 1964)*. This report was in the Dispensary No. 4 archives, suggesting Soviet authorities sought to compare notes on human radiation research in the United States.

given diagnoses in accordance with "state-sanctioned illnesses" like the flu or brucellosis.[32] Until the breakup of the Soviet Union in 1991, no official information or real medical assistance was offered to those examined by the dispensary's medical staff.

Neither the active nuclear testing nor the radioactive contamination impacted the grand new plan for the grasslands around Koian (which included certain sections of the Polygon). In 1953, a new Soviet leader, Nikita Khrushchev, embarked on what seemed at the time a brilliant solution to the Stalin-era grain crisis.[33] He proposed that the fragile "virgin" steppe grasslands, half of which are located in northern and central Kazakhstan, be transformed into gigantic agricultural farms. Khrushchev inaugurated the Virgin Lands campaign to significantly raise grain output to feed the nearly starving Soviet population in line with Soviet ideological goals: agricultural production could be and would be revolutionized along socialist lines. The vision of the future would be an efficient, integrated, and rational agro-industrial complex maintained by properly socialized Soviet bodies.[34] Concerns that Kazakhstan's grasslands were prone to wind and water erosion were dismissed and the Virgin Land campaign forged ahead at a swift "Sovietesque" tempo. Vast tracts of land – equal in size to the total cultivated area of Canada – were seeded with wheat and other cereals.[35]

From a purely economic standpoint, the kolkhoz was deemed inefficient at producing massive quantities of much-needed agricultural goods. As a result, colossal *sovkhozy* (state-owned farms) – long seen as an advanced form of socialist organization – were rapidly built from scratch or emerged from consolidated and less productive kolkhozy. Technoscientific animal breeding techniques (cross-breeding sheep and intensive livestock production) were introduced, which in turn further altered traditional Kazakh grazing practices. In various locations such as Koian, traditional free-range grazing techniques, often considered antiquated, were replaced with feedlots, leading to faster weight gain in animals. Machinery and workers were also sent to the region, even though settlers from European Russia already occupied the Kazakh steppe (including the Semipalatinsk area) in large numbers in the late nineteenth century.[36] Tens of thousands of tractors and other machinery arrived on trains in the Virgin Lands accompanied by hundreds of thousands of settlers to work these machines.[37] Khrushchev recruited workers by appealing to the ideological sensibilities of the Soviet youth, and over time they numbered in the hundreds of thousands. These were the unpaid, idealistic volunteer *Komsomol* (All-Union Leninist Young Communist League) brigades dispatched to *podnimat' tselinu* (raise the Virgin Lands). The new arrivals also included a large population of Stalin-era political deportees and prisoners, as well as individuals in search of work, an ethnically mixed group that included Russians, Ukrainians, Poles, Chechens, Tatars, Germans, and others.[38] In subsequent years, millions of students, soldiers, former prisoners from the gulag, and special settlers (mostly political deportees from Soviet Union's border regions) swelled the numbers further, establishing tent cities in the steppe and joining large grain and livestock sovkhozy.[39]

Similar to other sovkhozy in Kazakhstan, the Virgin Lands campaign in 1954 meant a near-immediate economic redevelopment for Koian.[40]

Its success, however, cannot be understood without considering the new village of Oktiabr' (October). As the story is told in Koian, a new settlement appeared "unexpectedly." "We just woke up one day and there were people building a new village," Burkut relayed during his interview. Hundreds of Russian and other non-Kazakh settlers spread out a tent colony on an open steppe some dozen kilometres away. In a matter of months, Oktiabr' had a neat grid pattern of cinder block homes, a school, administration buildings, a sports complex, a medical clinic, and even a graded secondary road.

The new village became the administrative arm of the region's burgeoning agro-industrial complex, and as a result Koian (because of its proximity) was utterly transformed from just a peripheral Kazakh kolkhoz to a "rurally cosmopolitan" agricultural node. Oktiabr' was designated the managerial and sovkhoz centre, while Koian and four other villages or *otdeleniia* (sectors) – along with at least fifty *zimovki* (winter settlements and pastures) – were assigned specific roles on the collective.[41] The otdeleniia were tasked with raising livestock and specialized in breeding cows, sheep, horses, and goats or combinations of these. Yields were shipped to Oktiabr' and then onward along a transport link in a long chain of distribution centres throughout Kazakhstan that delivered agricultural goods throughout the Soviet Union.

The life improvements that followed the Virgin Land campaign are remembered fondly by the older generation of Koianers. For them, the sovkhoz was idyllic yet modern, providing a sense of purpose. Before the end of 1955, all settlements within the sovkhoz had electricity, while additional housing, schools, medical clinics, and dormitories were constructed. Consumer goods became available and regular monthly wages allowed people to access previously unattainable goods. For the first time, locals could buy bicycles, building supplies, and food products. The well-maintained dirt road and bus service connecting Koian to Oktiabr' was particularly welcomed. For Burkut, life became much easier:

> We finally got glass windows, salaries, vacations, and real houses. Volunteers came to Koian, erected barns for livestock and then built cinder block houses, stores, and a dormitory. There was even a radio and telephone [available only at the administrative centre building]. When volunteers raised the Virgin Lands we had so much bread – we were still collecting the wheat harvest in December![42] Life really improved and we participated in the building of communism. Economically it was better then.

For most, the sovkhoz brought the socialist future that the Soviet leadership boasted about. Regardless of the bombs exploding in the distance, villagers like Burkut primarily remembered that the population grew and experienced an increase in the standard of living.

As local history is told, the Virgin Lands campaign hoisted Koian out of abject poverty. In 1954 the town's name was officially changed to Otdelenie (Sector) No. 4 and the village reorganized to raise thousands of sheep and horses, all kept on the territories of the eleven zimovki under its jurisdiction. "We had thousands of horses and sheep, while the sovkhoz produced a million tons of wheat per year. It's amazing how big our herds got! We also had technology – tractors, combines, lifts, and all sorts of machinery – electric scissors to shave sheep! Even Bulak zimovka had electricity," said Tursynbek. Each zimovka had at least two *chabany* (herders) who together with their extended families raised livestock. Some were even designed for Soviet youth brigades – a winter farm several kilometers from Bulak had a dormitory for a Komsomol brigade (at least fifty people). Enlisting for two years, individuals collectively raised thousands of sheep and goats for wool and meat. I spoke with Altynai and other women about the two years they spent in the Komsomol brigade. They described life in the zimovka as a time of freedom, when they made friends, found boyfriends, had fun, and became exemplary Soviet citizens rewarded for the hard work of helping the Soviet Union reach an ambitious goal of breeding fifty million sheep. "Not everyone was admitted to the Komsomol. We had to have good grades and pass entrance exams on Marx, Lenin, atheism, and so on. Only the best people were accepted," offered one attendee. Koian indeed became a modern village by the standards of the day.

Overall, the reordering of space that occurred in the 1950s was administered by various hierarchically positioned officials in charge of a six-thousand-strong workforce, including brigade leaders, tractor drivers, reapers, veterinarians, herders, grain harvesters, repairmen and teachers. This division of labour was designed to embody the highest form of socialist development, with all parts needing to work together to ensure that the sovkhoz operated like a well-oiled proletarian machine. By the early 1960s, villagers noted a significant influx of new migrants to the region outnumbering the ethnic Kazakhs, who found themselves a minority population on ancestral land. As elsewhere in Kazakhstan, most managerial roles in the sovkhoz were given to resettled Europeans, including Russians, Germans, and Ukrainians. Despite this inequality, the individuals I interviewed did not report any ethnic strife or tensions – in fact, just the opposite. Many people I spoke to in Koian and Oktiabr' remembered individuals from other nationalities favourably, especially Germans, who were seen as clean and precise and thus highly valued workers. It was only in the early 1990s, after the fall of the Soviet Union, that some Koianers began to report feeling resentment towards some Russians, whom they blamed for dismantling the sovkhoz and stealing formerly collective property.

While the Virgin Land campaign increased the overall grain output in the Soviet Union and is remembered as a grand period of history by many villagers, Western scholars have deemed it as an ultimately ecologically destructive example of the Soviet system.[43] Industrial-scale farming unleashed a barrage of effects on a landscape ill-equipped to handle the shock of such techniques. The problems quickly snowballed: failing to rotate crops while overgrazing delicate soils – coupled with a relentless pressure to boost output – soon led to catastrophic erosion. Dust Bowl–like conditions were reported in many parts of Kazakhstan.[44] At the same time, the poorly trained workforce with poorly researched methods set out with fertilizers, pesticides, and insecticides (beginning in the 1970s), applying these liberally while downplaying any environmental concerns.[45]

But the end of atomic testing and the dismantling of the sovkhoz system marked yet another turning point for the villagers. In a new paradoxical trade-off – capitalism and a nuclear-free existence in exchange for scarcity – the state effectively abandoned villagers to make do on their own. The collapse of the Soviet Union in 1991 marked a sudden wholesale transformation of the social, political, and economic orders in Kazakhstan that once again turned Koian into a periphery zone.[46]

After the Bombs

Scholars of post-socialist transformations generally agree that the end of the Soviet Union is not a uniform event.[47] Kazakhstan in general and Koian specifically represented an acute example of how this disintegration was localized and uniquely place specific.

Like elsewhere in Kazakhstan, the transformation of the Soviet command economy after 1991 was characterized by the "unraveling of the previously entwined character of Soviet work, domestic life, and the person."[48] By the mid-1990s, the sovkhoz was abandoned and a large class of dispossessed people began working with what was left. Systemic shortages of consumer goods and agricultural products were a standard part of Soviet existence, but the dismantling of the sovkhoz stripped Koianers of property, work, and social protections and divested them of their status.

Unlike large cities throughout the Soviet Union – Moscow, Leningrad, and Chelyabinsk – the rural areas saw the exodus of large numbers of people. In the first decade following the collapse, nearly all Ukrainians,

Belarusians, Germans, Poles, Tatars, and other Russian-speaking minorities left the sovkhoz, anxious about their future economic prospects in a state increasingly dominated by ethnic Kazakhs. They either resettled in large urban centres or departed Kazakhstan entirely to settle in their respective countries of origin. Ethnic Kazakhs also left en masse. Some families moved to the more populated Oktiabr' or opted for the burgeoning urban slums on the periphery of Karaganda or other large cities where family members had already established themselves.

The number of people who moved away is astonishing. In 1991, Koian had around seven hundred inhabitants; in 1999 the population dropped to just below two hundred; and in 2012, I counted fifty men, women, and children in total living in nine separate households – a number that still held in 2023. The numbers are similar for Oktiabr'. According to a local administrator with access to demographic statistics for the former sovkhoz administrative centre, all non-Kazakhs left save for one Tatar and one Russian. Before the Soviet collapse, the population of nearly three thousand residents in Oktiabr' had dwindled to barely nine hundred people by 2012.[49] To put the exodus in perspective, according to the Agency of the Republic of Kazakhstan on Statistics,[50] at the start of my fieldwork in 2010 in the Karaganda *oblast'* (administrative region), the majority of people lived in urban areas, with 77.5 per cent of people in the cities and 22.5 per cent in villages respectively.[51]

With the great out-migration, there are few explicit signs of the former non-Kazakh inhabitants. In a meadow located just outside of Oktiabr' lies a large, overgrown Christian cemetery where Russians, Germans, and others are buried in hardly identifiable plots. Aside from this spot, the once multi-ethnic landscape of the sovkhoz is lacking in objects through which the vibrant history could be narrated.

Accompanying the exodus, state oversight and the economic system disintegrated, leading to the collapse of the sovkhoz infrastructure. The road to ruin was short and exacerbated by the fact that people were not the only ones leaving the sovkhoz – they were taking whatever significant capital there was with them. Koianers not only lost their jobs, money, housing, and access to healthcare and education, but also watched in alarm as state property was plundered, taken by former sovkhoz administrators who were never seen again. Thousands of animals, tons of grain, countless tractors, combine harvesters, plows, trucks, and other industrial agriculture machinery *propalo* (vanished). Likewise, residential homes and other buildings were dismantled entirely – the *kirpich* (brick) was either reassembled elsewhere or sold at the market – adding to the landscape of ruins.

The period was often remembered as *repressiia* (repression), a term typically used to describe Stalin's brutal policies, but in this context a return to the "ancestral way of life" and a temporary loss of "civilization." As Burkut explained, "People did whatever they wanted – they took tractors and animals, and the smarter ones took both. The former sovkhoz directors, brigade leaders, and everyone else who worked in the upper administrative posts during the Soviet period took everything and moved away." The sovkhoz was plundered while the poorest of Koian residents watched in horror as their herds dwindled and food supply ran out. Seemingly overnight, the once celebrated animal herders, hay collectors, tractor drivers, and other labourers – the supposed backbone of the sovkhoz – became a class of rural poor. Their fates depended on the benevolence of former sovkhoz administrators who "allowed" them to keep a couple of cows, maybe a horse or two, a dozen sheep and goats, and one tractor to be shared among all residents of the entire sovkhoz.

"When the Soviet Union collapsed, life became unpredictable, and things here quickly turned to ruin," Tursynbek reminisced in the summer of 2015. The process of dismantling was catastrophic. In Koian, government infrastructure ground to a halt, and coal, diesel, electricity, food deliveries, bus service, emergency services, and road maintenance stopped.[52] In short order, Koian's food store, cafeteria, medical facility, and upper-grades school closed. There was no work and no cash income. Only in Oktiabr' could people obtain some limited goods – leftover medicines or grain. But because roads were inaccessible, people from Koian had to walk long distances to reach the former sovkhoz administrative centre. I listened again and again to stories of individuals who froze to death or were attacked by wolves outside the village as they walked through knee-deep snow from Koian to Oktiabr'.

Many stories I heard about the end of the Soviet Union centred on unexpected extreme financial hardships that resulted from the devaluation of the Russian ruble and the International Monetary Fund policy to shift the monetary system to the Kazakh tenge in 1993. While sawing a telephone pole for firewood, Tursynbek told me how in just one day he lost his entire life savings. If the loss of one's entire ideological structure was not enough, the financial collapse proved to be the last straw, utterly devastating to families in the village. With no resources and without the ability to self-manage the once promising collective, people survived the only way they knew how – on their diminished animal herds and on the new economy that developed on the Polygon.

Coinciding with the economic collapse of the region was the revelation of the impact of nuclear testing and the harmful effects of radiation exposure – information released under Mikhail Gorbachev's policies of *glasnost'* (openness).[53] This new move towards transparency provided a space for dialogue about previously undiscussed topics like media accounts of the 1986 Chornobyl (Chernobyl) disaster in Ukraine. Hearing from victims and seeing the media footage energized both local and global nuclear communities, and the Polygon and Chornobyl (Chernobyl) became a rallying point that led in time to a growing environmental crusade and the formation of the Nevada-Semipalatinsk antinuclear movement in Kazakhstan, headed by the Kazakh poet and intellectual Olzhas Suleimenov.[54] This international social-political activist organization, with the support of Nursultan Nazarbaev (the second in command of the Kazakh Soviet Socialist Republic), played a key role in ending nuclear testing.[55] It was during an attempted coup against Gorbachev that Nazarbaev officially "closed" the Polygon on August 29, 1991 – the forty-second anniversary of the first Soviet test.

Atomic Reflections

Historians and anthropologists alike have done a remarkable job in capturing Soviet modernization projects, their centralized economic planning, and the "ordinary life in extraordinary times" of Stalin's terrorized Russia.[56] But places like Koian are rarely written into the grand narrative account of Soviet history. In part this is because Koian's story begins at the margins of the Tsarist Empire, then shifts to the margins of the Soviet state, only to continue at the margins of present-day Kazakhstan. Yet it offers a remarkable case study within a larger recognizable history – a place with its own distinctiveness, but nevertheless one emblematic of the Soviet shared experience. Koian was at the centre of some of the most dramatic transformations ever to take place on Kazakh soil. How individuals were incorporated by the Soviet Union is reflected in the stories people tell, and the Bolshevik Revolution was the beginning of the end for the Kazakh traditional way of life. Yet inside what became the secretive military zone, people in Koian were socially and economically sustained by the Soviet system. Everyone had access to better food products, free healthcare (however limited), education, job training, and a guarantee that the next generation of Soviet citizens would be provided for. This sustenance, however, came at a price. The Cold War arms race, resulting in the intensification of nuclear testing and the Virgin Lands campaign, subjected communities to multiple sources of dangerous contaminants in a single site, or what anthropologists Donna Goldstein and Kira Hall[57] call "toxic layering."[58] Since the collapse of the Soviet Union, Western scholarship has gone to great lengths to uncover the damage left behind. Kazakhstan in particular features prominently in narratives about ecological ruin with the Aral Sea desiccation, the Virgin Lands campaign's soil erosion, and the fallout from nuclear testing on the Polygon.[59] The villages in and around the Polygon are some of the most neglected and impoverished areas in the country, and there is near-uniform agreement among spectators that the site is an ecological disaster (I say near-uniform because curiously absent from the post-Soviet history are the thoughts and viewpoints of the local villagers, who have a remarkably different attitude towards their home and the impacts of radiation on it).

Despite the predominant interpretive framework of Soviet "ecocide" in scholarly literature, Koianers in my study neither saw the Virgin Lands campaign nor nuclear testing in the region as spawning an environmental catastrophe. As noted by historians Laurent Coumel and Marc Elie,[60] the ecocide literature "does nothing to advance further understanding of both the real place of nature within the Soviet project and the weight of impact of environmental sensibilities in the population."

Zhanbolat was one of a few individuals who saw the beginning and the end of the Soviet era in Koian, and his remarks are reflective of the attitudes of many Koianers when looking back on its nuclear past and forward into a radioactive future. He was one of three elder residents in Koian when I met him in November 2010. My visit came two weeks after his seventieth birthday and one week after his release from the hospital. When we met that November, he was visibly suffering – stomach cancer had appeared suddenly and there were no drugs to manage the pain, so doctors prescribed him aloe tea. However, this was not his first time dealing with a serious illness. In 2004, a large malignant tumour was surgically removed from his right eye, leaving behind a three-inch scar.

Like his parents and grandparents before him, Zhanbolat was born in Koian and prided himself on never having moved away. After finishing primary school there in the mid-1950s, he took on many occupations in what was to be a lifelong career on the collective farm: a tractor driver, sheepherder, hay and grain collector, as well as an accountant. Zhanbolat had ten children (four girls and six boys, the youngest of whom was twenty-one years old), a feat that earned his wife the Soviet honorary title of "Mother Heroine."[61] In 2006, she unexpectedly died from tongue cancer when she was only in her fifties. I would soon learn that in the Polygon region, people rarely lived long enough to see retirement pensions and that surviving past fifty is a blessing. Zhanbolat, therefore, belonged to a very small group of *stariki* (elders), a handful of individuals who reached old age in these parts of Kazakhstan. Even for his advanced age (or perhaps because of it), he was determined to report to me the "truth about the Polygon's past and present." Yet his truth departed in important ways from the accepted Western narrative:

> After each test, the commanders gave 150 grams of vodka to the soldiers. They gave us nothing! We were experimental rabbits, but we didn't know that then! But now, my body is adapted to radiation and if I leave, I will either get sick or die. Clean air is our death, so we can't leave. And of course, we worked here and on the Polygon – we cut hay, harvested grain, and grazed sheep, everything ... there was no fence and everyone went where they were told to go or wanted to go. In those times, what is radiation, how dangerous it is, we did not know. They knew, we didn't know, and now we are used to it. Everyone was afraid to give a real diagnosis. For example, if someone was sick from radiation, some doctors probably knew, but couldn't tell us because they risked arrest. So instead, they gave a fake diagnosis and that's it. You couldn't openly say that people were sick from radiation because it was a secret ...
>
> A lot of people were shot or arrested by the NKVD [a Soviet government agency that functioned as the secret police and served as a forerunner to the KGB] in Koian for not following the law, but that was only because of Stalin. For example, one of my family members hid in the Tsarist mine to avoid going to war. The NKVD officers tied his mother to a pole, threatening to shoot her if he did not come out. He did – they arrested him and he died somewhere in the war, but we don't know where. But after Stalin we had everything: money, coal, and hay. Everything was cheap. We had vacations and life wasn't bad. You get used to the bombs.

Zhanbolat's descriptions of his experiences touch on many aspects of daily life in Koian during this period. On the one hand, people who lived in the zone are not afraid to express their current anxiety about radiation exposure and are bitter that for forty years they knew nothing about what was going on. On the other hand, life in the Polygon required adaptation to the conditions at hand, and as Zhanbolat points out, it followed the rhythms of the collective farm and not so much those of testing. Couples got married. Children went to school. Adults were preoccupied with livestock herding, hay and grain harvesting, and other farm duties. Hence the secret nuclear tests, a regular sight in Koian, just became a normal interruption. When it all ended, life in Koian became harder once again, leading Zhanbolat in his remaining years to yearn for a better time (he died in 2013 from cancer).[62]

I heard similar stories from others. Nurzhan, who was born in Koian and in her mid-sixties, was just a child when she suffered from what she now believes was radiation sickness. She spoke to me about her experience at a clinic where she now works as a physician:

> I was five or six years old when the bomb exploded – it must have been 1962. By looking directly at the light I was blinded and developed cataracts. Then there were these strange burns on my body that made my skin peel. All my hair fell out. Without available transportation, my parents couldn't take me to the hospital, so I stayed in bed for months instead. There was a Polish doctor in Koian. He was a victim of Stalin's repressions and very happy not to end up in one of the notorious labour camps. He tried to heal everyone, even though he lacked drugs. He helped me. But no one ever gave me a diagnosis – the doctor probably didn't know himself what was going on. Because I am a doctor now and finally learned what was happening in Koian when these tests took place, I am certain that it was radiation sickness. But it's hard to be mad. We fed the Soviet nation and were provided with all the necessities of life. I was a doctor here in the sovkhoz. But our parents never had to think about how they are going to provide for us – the state did it for them. People shouldn't criticize the Soviet Union. I worked for the Soviet authorities and there were never any problems – to get stuck outside of the aul? Never! We always had a road that was maintained. We had a sea of plows, a sea of tractors – even Bulak [a winter farm] had them. We did not have to think about tomorrow – we lived for today.

Residents, the media, or the authorities publicly never mentioned radiation or elements like strontium, caesium, plutonium, and countless others known to cause illness and death with repeated exposure.[63] In fact, until the late 1980s the use of the term *radiatsiia* (radiation) was officially forbidden and an unfamiliar term to residents. In effect, the "illegality" of certain words made proper medical diagnoses impossible, and Nurzhan was not familiar with the term until much later. Even a cancer diagnosis was illegal, and in official documents these deaths often appear as heart attacks, aneurisms, or other unrelated diseases. For Nurzhan, her deep connections to the Soviet past reveal an additional level of complexity. Although she believes she was exposed to radioactive fallout, she is not angry but rather is a proud former Soviet citizen who expected the government to modernize the economy and provide economic welfare in exchange for her political loyalty and hard work.[64] She believed she was able to become a physician and was guaranteed a job in the sovkhoz because her parents belonged to the Communist

Party. Even though not everyone had access to a university education like Nurzhan, everyone belonging to the sovkhoz was provided free occupational training, schooling, and healthcare.

There are several reasons for Zhanbolat's and Nurzhan's complex outlook that have roots in both Soviet-era history for Koianers and the post-Soviet world they are forced to navigate. It is clear that at the time nuclear testing was ongoing it was a well-guarded state secret that Koianers hardly knew anything about, and this is especially true with regard to radiation danger. There was no radiation to bemoan because no one knew it existed.[65] Unlike in the Soviet Union's plutonium-producing city of Ozersk, where the working classes were attracted by middle-class prosperity to live with residual radioactivity and health risks,[66] Koianers first learned about their local toxic legacy only in the late 1980s, when the Nevada-Semipalatinsk antinuclear movement in Kazakhstan made this information public.

Another key reason for the Koianers' seeming embrace of "ecocide" was that until the fall of the Soviet Union in 1991, they spent their lives within a collective system that offered them a better standard of living than they had before.[67] Typical was the experience of Altynai, who worked in a Komsomol brigade during the sovkhoz era at Koian. She told me that they did not have time to think about the environment or wait for the bombs to explode: "We were happy, we worked, and we had a normal life. The state provided us with all the necessities and the testing that went on was a brief interruption of our daily routines. No one knew that the bombs were radioactive." Remarks like this are not simply a case of nostalgic yearnings or a "romance with one's own fantasy."[68] The bucolic and idyllic stories Koianers tell about the period of the sovkhoz today are not reverent contemplation about a life that never was but rather a reflection of how their lives did actually improve. Since the Soviet disintegration, much has changed. Their status as respected citizens is gone, and their skill sets – perfect for a collective – have become unsuited to a market economy or completely useless. Unsurprisingly, many would like to see the test site reopened for their own commercial and private usage.

Conclusion

Unlike Zhanbolat, Erzhan spent most of his life tending animals inside the official borders of the Polygon, living in Bulak on a winter farm. He was born before World War II in a village located about twenty miles (about thirty kilometres) from Koian and was quickly orphaned. Locals say the NKVD murdered his parents for being "enemies of the state," but Erzhan did not go into details about this (though he did mention that both of his sisters were interned and died in a labour camp during the war). Adopted by "people," Erzhan moved to the winter farm in 1947, where he worked and lived for fifty years together with his wife and children. It is now a well-known fact that Bulak is toxic – indeed, it is located in one of the more radioactive sections of the Polygon, next to several technical areas used for underground nuclear testing. No less than twenty-three of these tests were conducted here, three of which were excavation explosions generating craters. The nearest of these craters is visible from the winter farm where he once lived:

We worked right in the centre of the Polygon, all around ground zero where they did the explosions. Before each test, a medical doctor from Moscow whose name was Biriukov (I forgot his patronymic) would come to the zimovka and warn us. He looked after us, a very nice man. Biriukov would tell us where to take our sheep so that they are safe from the blast and made sure we are safe too ... He would come during every test – a plane would make circles above making sure no one was left behind ... They prepared for these tests for six months so that everything is done perfectly without an accident. Biriukov would load us onto a bus and drive everyone to safety. He always had a special *preparat* [a liquid solution] that we had to drink. If there was no preparat, we drank vodka. And if there was no vodka, he told us to take 150 grams of sugar with water and drink that. He really helped us.

When I lived in the zimovka, we herded our animals, oh I don't know, two or three kilometres from the underground crater ... We absolutely knew nothing about radiation, no one told us that radiation can make people ill. But our organism is different now – we are used to it probably. For example, it turns out that right next to the zimovka they tested a neutron bomb! It was a poorly made bomb, so it poisoned everything as we later found out ... but we never got ill. The other craters were okay – there are fish there – you can still see a volleyball court and a diving board once used by soldiers. We lived close to the crater but never got sick. Why? Because we knew how to stay safe. For example, we ate horsemeat. As you know, horses generally don't have mutations and neither do mountain goats. I knew this because whenever I took my animals to pasture next to the crater, I saw plenty of two-headed or one-eyed mice. Sheep, goats, and cows also had these same mutations, but that's because all are biologically weak organisms. But I never saw mutations in horses or mountain goats! Also, the administrators helped us stay healthy. They brought us all sorts of fruits from Czechoslovakia, a country with strict food safety protocols. All fruits, for example, were kept in a refrigerator for six months and then they were tested in a laboratory. Radiation didn't affect us then, maybe now it does, but how would we even know?

We are sick – heart problems, skin problems, all sorts of problems. But maybe we didn't die because we can't live without it [radiation]. I recently drove by Bulak on my way to Semipalatinsk [Semey]. Scary how we lived is such a backward place. But at least then everything was green; now, the grass and soil look strange. In winter, the grass is so poisonous that it melts the snow.[69] You have to know that when we lived on the Polygon we had very good relations with soldiers and all administrators. Everyone visited us: doctors, commanders, lieutenants, and even generals ... commander Gerasimov is now in Moscow ... They really respected us, and we were the only ones they allowed to move freely on the Polygon. I didn't need authorization! On my motorcycle I went everywhere, even to Kurchatov when it was still a closed city. But the Russians should have cleaned up the Polygon and covered all the radiation with quality cement.

Erzhan's experiences of life on the Polygon are not structured around what may look like from the outside as a "state of emergency," as described by Walter Benjamin,[70] characterized by pervasive militarization of daily life, secrecy, and the blatant denial that anything was wrong. Quite the opposite. For him it was a pleasant kind of paternalism. Moreover, his story brings together what is nearly always kept separate in historiographies of the Polygon and the Virgin Lands campaign. These were not neatly separate undertakings, located in their own bounded space, but rather took shape on an overlapping landscape. The Polygon was not an uninhabited place for nuclear testing, nor were the people outside its borders victims. Accordingly, Erzhan's narrative challenges the erasure of a multiplicity of place-based cultural, political, and economic realities.[71] It also remarkably contradicts much of what is said about nuclear victims. Erzhan's description of life on the Polygon privileges the history of the Virgin Lands over that of nuclear testing, survival over trauma, and the porous nature of borders over their impermeability.

Most people I spoke with remember the sovkhoz life during atomic testing as pleasant and one that gave purpose and meaning to their existence. Even when people were told the "truth" – that they were exposed to radioactivity, were lied to, and were subject to medical radiation research – this information did not dislodge their ideas about the "good life." It is not to say that people who live in Koian and Oktiabr' are unaware of what happened to them, delude themselves through stories of pleasant sovkhoz life, or necessarily yearn for the past and the bombs. Rather, the stories they tell about their past reflect the fact that their lives during the Soviet years (especially after Stalin's death) were much improved. People had careers with paid vacations, enough food to eat, free medical care, and education. It could also be that the disruption and the misery of the post-Soviet years made Koianers reappraise their Soviet experience.

Today Koianers are no longer part of grandiose plans. They lack economic security, respectability, and status. And like before, they are at the centre of scientific debates about the effects of radiation but are not included in the conversation. Russian, Kazakh, and Western scientists continue to do research on the Polygon populations and don't share their findings. As Tursynbek often said to me, "We are once again traditional Kazakhs – nomads living in the steppe – and still experimental rabbits." Nurzhan expressed this anxiety to me too. She is uncertain as to what is really happening to the Polygon populations. In an offhanded way, she told me that perhaps people can't live in clean air or maybe simply that people don't want to leave the village because of the "Kazakh mentality" that keeps people tied to ancestral lands. Whatever the truth is, Nurzhan knows that many people died and continue to die from cancer, that animals were born with three or five legs or one eye, and that women gave birth to "gelatin" babies that had their organs on the outside. Whether these illnesses and tragedies were all radiation-related, she does not know. Nurzhan's medical expertise has led her to conclude that the only thing people can do now is to eat enough fruits and vegetables to at least make their bodies stronger.

2 "Clean Air Is Our Death": Debates about Genetic Mutation

Now hear this Earth! I am Mutant Man, Homo Superior! I have been created by radiation forces out of the loins of you, the human race, after your great terrible Atom Wars. Yes, I am a step up and beyond you, and I am now your master for better or worse. You created me in your blind, savage, senseless war of atomic radiation. You have only your-selves to blame if I turn out to be your – Frankenstein Monster!

– Otto Binder, "How Nuclear Radiation Can Change Our Race."
Mechanix Illustrated, December 1953

Introduction

In early fall, stockbreeders in Koian begin cutting and piling the tall steppe grasses. When the howling winds and deep snows come and the road disappears, their rickety barns full of sheep, cows, and horses will sag under its weight. It's early October 2010. I stand with Ramazan, Tursynbek's elder brother, on a small hill above the village and we look out upon a scene that's begun to frighten him. The grasses in the distance are burning. Although the fire had smoldered for days, one morning – two months into my twelve-month period of fieldwork – the flames began to rage. Smoke billowed in the distance, the skies darkened and the fire line spread, drawing closer to the village after dusk.

In this arid steppe, fires are common events that threaten the income and livelihood of the residents. The seemingly random placement of haystacks that dot the landscape and fuelled the blaze aren't in fact random at all. Koianers selectively harvest from the once Soviet agricultural fields of wheat and other grasses – plots that some of the older residents had worked while nuclear testing was occurring simultaneously.

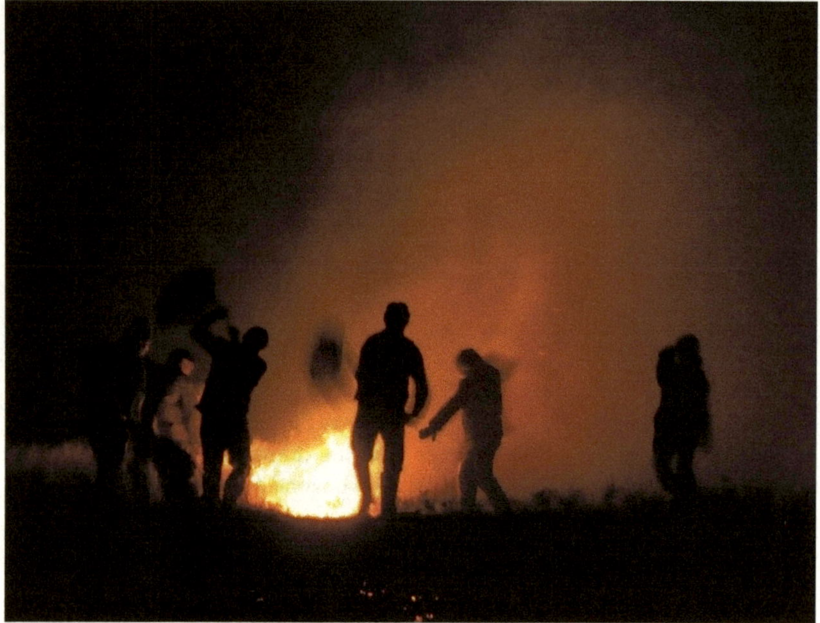

Figure 2.1. *Fire Brigade.* Men using long poles with sheepskins attached to extinguish a steppe fire.

Earlier that day on an otherwise clear morning save for the rising columns of smoke, at Ramazan's insistence we drove across the fields towards the fire line to assess the damage in the only functioning large car the village had: my old Mitsubishi Delica van. Ramazan complained that during the Soviet period, there had been fire crews and trucks, the likes of which could have helped. Luckily, one of the villagers had bartered for diesel, either from a mine where they pick shifts or from a neighbouring village. As we reached a small hill, we could see the grass steadily burning in all directions. High winds lifted embers, carrying them everywhere. Others were scanning the damage and preparing to act. The only priority was preventing a repeat of the previous year when an entire herd of some one hundred cows belonging to two families starved to death for lack of food. In a region where water is scarce and there is no fire department, we began to fight the blazes in the only way possible – by snuffing them out with rough-cut sheepskins attached to long poles.

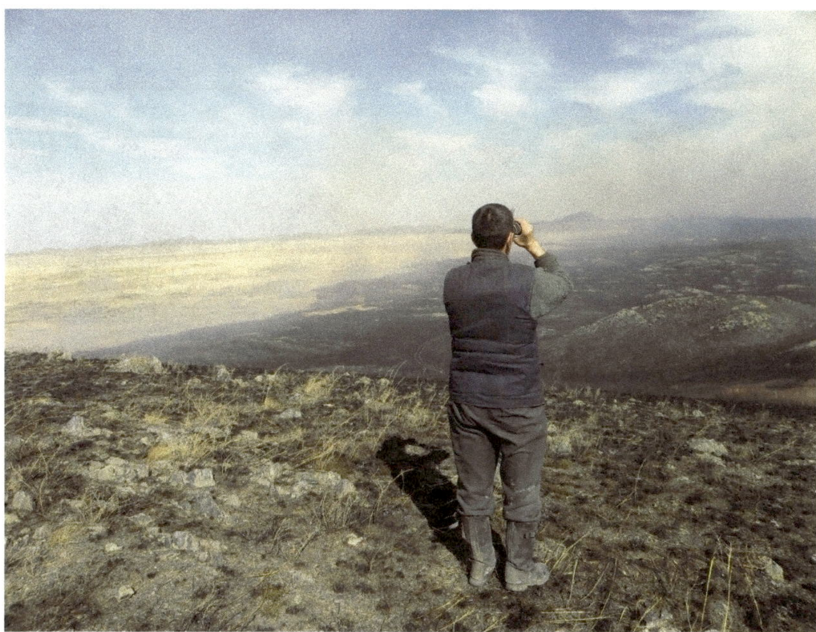

Figure 2.2. *Scorched Steppe*. The steppe fire burned through the Polygon. Koianers regularly inspected the extent of the damage that smoldered for weeks.

We packed the car with steel milk drums and, sloshing water all over, drove from one fire line to the next late into the night. The Delica had been transformed into a fire truck.

Although our fire brigade seemed effective, I was scared for another reason. This blaze, only the first of 2010, would pass right through the nuclear test site. This was when I realized that its boundaries, represented clearly on a map hanging in my one-room house in Koian, meant absolutely nothing. Neither fire nor radioactive particles obey borders. Every time we hit the flame with our sheepskins or ran through the charred earth towards the next fire line with buckets full of water hoisted from a well, we crossed in and out of the old atomic site. But no one really knew when because there were no signs or fences to warn us. I imagined radioactive particles – buried somewhere in layers of ash – re-suspended in the air once again, covering our clothes and being drawn into our lungs.

For four days we chased and battled a blaze that burned the test site in lines stretching to the horizon.

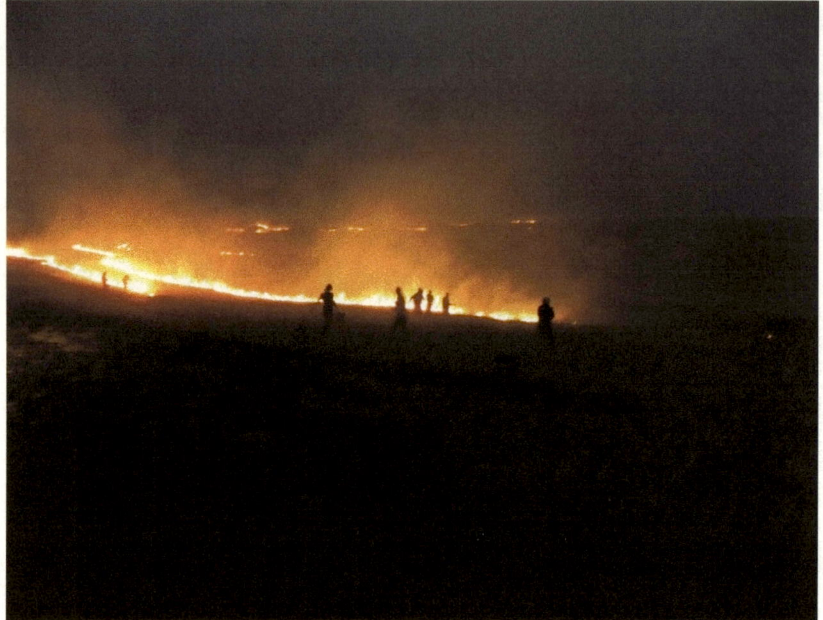

Figure 2.3. *Fire Line.* The steppe fire burned in lines stretching to the horizon. Men and women from Koian worked to extinguish a rapidly spreading grass fire near their village.

Paradoxically, the general attitude wasn't one of fear or anger but rather one of simultaneous excitement and annoyance. We spoke about saving the haystacks, about how the government couldn't care less about "backward" rural *aul'skie* (villagers) who didn't deserve their own fire brigade, and how in this seemingly isolated part of the Kazakh steppe, the fire looked pretty, resembling city lights glowing at night in the distance.

We also laughed about how easily I lost my way in the dark and how alien I looked donning a sanitary mask that I had bought in a pharmacy months earlier and encouraging others to do the same. But throughout it all, not once did anyone mention or even seem concerned about the smoke rising from areas where radioactive caesium-137, strontium-90, plutonium-239, and other transuranic elements are known to exist in hotspots.[1] No one seemed concerned that the fire travelled through craters from underground nuclear explosions and some of the most toxic aboveground nuclear tests, only to stop – nearly a month later – more than seventy miles (more than one hundred kilometres) away at Kurchatov.

During the fire, I wondered about the villagers' seeming lack of fear or anger. After all, everyone knew that living next to the nuclear test site meant that radiation exposure was likely – not only during fires but whenever people travelled through the territory proper to visit relatives in other settlements or to collect wild berries. My Geiger counter acted as a set of eyes and ears, allowing me to "see" and "hear" radiation – the tasteless, odourless, and invisible harm emanating from the ground beneath my feet. But over time it became burdensome and even embarrassing to scan the ground everywhere I went. Early in my fieldwork, I constantly thought of things to scan: shoes, clothes, car tires, random pieces of concrete and metal strewn about the village, and even house walls, both inside and out. Although it's frantic clicking regularly indicated the presence of radioactive elements, most people preferred to avoid me instead because they thought I suffered from excessive paranoia. At some point, the Geiger counter became a sort of electronic intruder, forcing people to think about radiation in a place where no one thought about it in day-to-day life. But I remained puzzled: how can radiation be the least of people's problems?

What came into view for me during this particular fire and the subsequent visits to the region was this: although Koian residents have much in common with other "radiogenic communities"[2] near nuclear weapons test sites and the so-called peaceful nuclear industries (such as uranium mining), they have a complicated relationship with and have in part *embraced* radiation and turned it into a virtue. In defining themselves this way, they challenged the hegemony of "nuclear victimhood" and what some anthropologists have come to understand as biomedical "ideologies of health."[3] *Victim* among Polygon residents meant "deprived of agency" – which they are not. Instead, they saw their lives and those of their children as proof of a locally specific form of adaptation. They often told me when we travelled through the Polygon that *"my privykli k radiatsii"* (we are used to radiation).

Locals told and retold narratives imbued with this particular kind of certainty regarding radiation, helping people make sense of their lives and justify their existence. Forced to venture more than one hundred miles (about 150 kilometres) to the nearest grocery store to buy monthly supplies, they would report headaches, dizziness, and stomach cramps while outside the village, but the symptoms would vanish when they returned home. Typical were remarks shared one afternoon by Burkut, the oldest man in the village, as he sat on a large disintegrating Soviet tractor tire:

> Our organism is different. What we eat is poisonous. But we eat only food that is well cooked – boiled or grilled – so that radiation can evaporate, at least a little. But our organism is now accustomed to radiation. For many years we were exposed to radioactive fallout, and now we eat it. Slowly and quietly, our bodies got used to it. Why do you think people don't die in Koian but only get a little sick? Those who move to the city away from Koian can survive only for a maximum of two years. Many people moved away to start new lives in the city, and only two individuals out of that large group are still alive. Why? It's simple. Most of us can't live in clean air – we need radiation to survive. Clean air is our death.

This is not to say that they didn't see themselves as casualties of the Soviet military complex,[4] suffering from chronic ailments like skin rashes, high blood pressure, heart problems, and cancers, which they link to past and present radioisotope exposure. But unlike the survivors of the Chornobyl (Chernobyl) disaster in Ukraine, who use claims of damaged biology to access limited state resources,[5] residents near the Semipalatinsk Test Site "embraced" radiation and the "slow violence"[6] it engenders as a sign of their own genetic adaptation. By this they meant not only that they could survive it but also that it *helped* them stay alive; others who had left, they said, died as a result. Burkut, Tursynbek, and others warned that if I stayed long, I too might come to "depend on radiation."

The Debate about Low-Dose Radiation

Far away from the Polygon for the past two decades in Kazakhstan's scientific circles (and even longer in the West), a debate has raged concerning low-dose radiation and pathological genetic change. Despite nearly a century of scientific research on the long-term biological effects of low-dose radiation, nuclear science is a form of "partial knowledge,"[7] with many unanswered questions that may or may not have implications for long-term public health. Since the bombing of Hiroshima and Nagasaki in 1945, radioactive products have been steadily released across the globe, yet the human risks remain poorly understood and little has been settled. Notwithstanding the testing programs of the United States, the Soviet Union, France, and Britain, and the studies of non-combat-related events like Three Mile Island, Chornobyl (Chernobyl), and Fukushima, there is a general sense of uncertainty and anxiety among researchers and the millions of people across the world (the "global hibakusha") exposed to radiation about long-term radiation and health outcomes.[8]

The partial knowledge regarding radiation is reflected in the concept of low-dose radiation itself, defined by the US National Academy of Sciences as an amount equal to background-level radiation and below which health effects are undetectable.[9] As a result, it is, by definition, near impossible to link chronic ailments with diseases like cancers of the lung and oesophagus that are geographically associated with high-risk areas. Although these cancers may indeed result from radiation exposure – especially if the high-risk area is a nuclear test site – their decades-long latency period (from exposure to symptom) makes it nearly impossible to determine whether a particular toxicant (tobacco, alcohol, radiation) or lifestyle (diet or lack of exercise) is responsible:

> There is little doubt that people living in the STS [Semipalatinsk Test Site] region suffer from a range of adverse health effects ... However, the task of definitely relating any of these effects to nuclear weapons testing will be complicated by numerous confounding factors such as inadequate nutrition, poor water quality, and unsanitary living conditions.[10]

As the anthropologist S. Lochlann Jain points out, cancer is a "set of relationships – economic, sentimental, medical, personal, ethical, institutional, statistical" – and therefore not solely reducible to "a biological phenomenon."[11] This multilayered context makes it difficult to clearly connect cause and effect,[12] and since radiation exposure is a global phenomenon, finding "virgin" populations to serve as control groups is impossible.[13]

Although the National Research Council[14] has concluded that low-dose radiation and illness cannot be clearly linked, scientists generally agree that there is no threshold below which radiation exposure produces zero effect. They also agree that humans are the most radiation-resistant mammal.[15] While any amount of radiation exposure poses some health risks, the generally accepted scientific position is that there are no data that show lifetime radiation doses below 10,000 millirem cause cancer or any other illnesses.[16] Yet a key difficulty in establishing causality between radiation exposure and illness lies with temporality. The "slow violence"[17] that radiation exposure in low doses tends to engender – chronic illnesses such as lung, thyroid, stomach, or other cancers, for example – frequently appears years or even decades after exposure and depends upon multiple factors, from exposure rates to personal genetics to the types of radionuclides present in the environment.[18]

Plutonium, for example, stays mostly in place and can be stopped by a sheet of paper, but is dangerous when inhaled; tritium is easily transported with underground water; and strontium-90, a "bone seeker," behaves very much like calcium and is easily absorbed by plants and deposits in the bone tissue and bone marrow of animals.[19] Migration of radionuclides is also a dynamic process: an area may be clean one day but become contaminated the next.

Although low-dose radiation could be dangerous, there is no evidence that exposure to it causes congenital anomalies, chromosomal aberrations, or any other cellular abnormalities among adult populations. More important, the consensus has it that genetic damage caused by radiation cannot be passed on to offspring. In biomedicine, *genetic mutation* refers to a permanent change in the DNA sequence that results in a new reproductive outcome. Such a mutation can be either inherited from a parent (known as a germ-line mutation, since it occurs in the germ cells, ova and sperm) or acquired during a person's life (known as a somatic mutation). According to the Radiation Effects Research Foundation,

> Detection of human germ cell mutations is difficult, especially at low doses. While high doses in experimental animals can cause various disorders in offspring (birth defects, chromosome aberrations, etc.), no evidence of clinical or subclinical effects has yet been seen in children of A-bomb survivors.[20]

These conclusions are grounded in the longitudinal studies of atomic bomb survivors from Hiroshima and Nagasaki, considered the gold standard in radiation science. However, the studies themselves tend to minimize the possibility of harm[21] by excluding data on risks from low-dose exposure associated with inhaling or ingesting radioactive elements that can lodge in the body and irradiate cells indefinitely.[22] At the same time, the view of them as the gold standard is partly a Cold War political phenomenon, in which scientists have elevated US–Japanese data as a way to discredit their Soviet counterparts.[23] For this reason, the Western scientific radiological establishment often dismisses or critiques as not rigorous those studies that contradict it[24] – studies that, for example, find that radiation causes serious mutations in the germ line even in low doses and that somatic mutations are, in fact, transmittable.[25]

In the Soviet Union and the post-Soviet states like Kazakhstan or Ukraine, the biological effects of radiation exposure are understood differently and contradict the gold standard studies. During the Cold

War, the secrecy surrounding the Soviet atomic project prevented researchers from discussing radiation and conducting public-safety risk assessments. As historian Kate Brown[26] explains, unlike their US counterparts, Soviet scientists lacked access to even the most rudimentary data on the types and amounts of radioisotopes released into the environment. This information was classified. While US researchers could track them in the environment – linking them to quantifiable and singular physical effects, such as thyroid cancer – Soviet researchers were obliged to observe, trace, and decode minute changes in blood cells and organs, in bone composition, and in physical and mental aptitude.[27] They linked concurrent symptoms, such as anaemia, chronic fatigue, joint pain, nosebleeds, and brittle bones to biological changes and subsequently to what they called chronic radiation syndrome (CRS). Yet despite fifty years of data on CRS and research on the biogenetic effects of low-dose radiation more broadly, Western scientists still dismiss Soviet and post-Soviet findings as politically and ideologically tainted.[28]

Radiophobia as a Discursive Strategy

Since 1993, the Institute of Radiation Safety and Ecology (IRSE) in Kurchatov, under the direction of the NNC, has overseen the Polygon. Lacking both the funds and means to secure the site, it collects data on commercial activities in highly contaminated but unmarked areas. The IRSE estimates that eighty zimovki in the region are used "illegally" for breeding some thirty thousand sheep, four thousand cows, and three thousand horses, as well as for other forms of agricultural production[29] while residents also occasionally find work mining coal, manganese, fluorite, gold, or other minerals. The IRSE detected elevated but not "dangerous" levels of strontium-90, plutonium-239, and plutonium-240 in these pastures' grasses and other plants, as well as in the bones and soft tissues of stock animals.[30] The Institute explicitly disallows small-scale stockbreeding because of health risks, yet they go on unregulated.

In recent years the IRSE has been promoting a new economic plan to "hoist the region out of poverty" in the words of the former deputy director general for radioecology – a wider project designed to eventually privatize most of the roughly seven-thousand-square-mile (about eighteen-thousand-square-kilometre) Polygon. The Institute aims to properly secure the most radioactive areas of the test site, then set aside 90 per cent of the territory for industrial agriculture, livestock breeding, and mining operations. Supported by the International Atomic Energy Agency, the plan aims to promote an inhabited, economically viable radioactive landscape.[31] At the same time, Kazakhstan's political leadership has accelerated its long-term economic development agendas focused on extractive industries (e.g., Kazakhstan 2020, 2030, and 2050). In 2014, several agencies were merged into one Ministry of Energy, including the Ministry of the Environment and Water Resources (in charge of managing natural resources and environmental hazards) and the Ministry of Industry and New Technologies (responsible for nuclear safety). These new bureaucracies are industry forward, promoting green energy (including nuclear power generation), natural resource extraction, and environmental protection.

According to many critics who oppose development plans for the region[32] – including a former deputy director of IRSE, together with numerous medical doctors, non-governmental organization (NGO) workers, and government officials – the data meant to prove that the Polygon is safe have been cherry picked. They accused the promoters of the plan of advancing an *antiobshchestvennoi* (antisocial) program: in their view deliberately minimizing risk and ignoring radiation danger bordered on criminal negligence and careless risk taking with the health of hundreds of thousands of people. Worse, by attempting to privatize economic activities that were already taking place in unmarked and contaminated areas of the Polygon, the plan's advocates sought to end debate on the issue of residual radioactivity and the legacies of environmental and human health. Instead of debate, large mining corporations and members of Kazakhstan's political elite were investing heavily in the area and did not want their products associated with radioactivity. Official plans to develop the test site coincide with broader governmental interests in expanding its nuclear energy program and extracting uranium for Western markets.

What happened next reflects the curious legacy of Soviet nuclear toxicity. As anthropologist Catherine Alexander[33] observes, "There are sometimes insurmountable tensions in the state-building exercises of securing both a particular version of the nuclear past on Kazakh land, and nuclear futures as a distinctively Kazakh enterprise." These tensions, in turn, have come to shape the Institute's ability to "reconfigure its relationship with the STS [the Polygon] and move forward."[34] The "integral part of the process of moving on," Alexander argues, is contingent upon "particular ways of knowing"[35] the site and controlling the discourse about its toxic legacies. The Institute plays a key role in producing scientific information about the test site, but it also controls a discursive space – who gets to talk about it, how, when, and where. Matters concerning residual radioactivity are physically and discursively regulated, and Institute officials see discussions about radiation residue and ill health as leaving the country mired in Soviet legacies of nuclear toxicity. They are of the opinion that the Polygon is generally safe and poses no danger to human health unless people access contaminated areas for extended periods. Therefore, the acceptable way of viewing fear of radioactive toxicity and public health is as a societal-level problem the Institute has to address through education and "psychological normalization" – not environmental remediation of the Polygon.[36] To encourage this view, it recently has promoted awareness-raising community outreach programs designed to combat *radiophobia*.

Radiophobia was first recognized by science experts and industry specialists after the 1986 Chornobyl (Chernobyl) disaster in Ukraine to describe public reaction considered out of proportion to the real risk of the accident.[37] These experts claimed that the majority of health problems (anxiety, depression, fevers, stomach aches, headaches, suicide, and so on) among survivors of the disaster were due to irrational fear.[38] As a psychological disorder, radiophobia gathered legitimacy when the Chernobyl Forum,[39] a consortium of United Nations agencies and nuclear industry experts, scientifically evaluated the human and environmental consequences of the disaster. It argued that the primary radiation-related illness that would be noticeable was the mostly treatable thyroid cancer, which was especially pronounced among exposed children.

As one of the top experts at the Institute explained during an interview with me in 2012, "Whereas other parts of the world are blessed with palm trees, mild weather, and sandy beaches, Kazakhstan has a wealth of natural resources, especially uranium, and naturally radioactive environments instead. There are tens of thousands of radioactive sources in the country. Radiation is part of Kazakhstan's landscape and has always been." He went on to explain that radiophobia is actually a much bigger problem than radioactive contamination. Because radiation is invisible, he continued, it has become an "ideal enemy" and a perfect "scapegoat" for people like those living around the Polygon who lead "risky" lives by consuming too much tobacco and alcohol. In his view, they would rather blame radiation for their ill health then change their otherwise "irresponsible behaviour."

Complicating matters is the fact that toxicity in and around the Polygon has played a key role in post-Soviet nation building. One of the first decrees by Kazakh President Nursultan Nazarbaev in 1991 was to close the Soviet nuclear test site and go public with the nuclear tragedy. These actions required detailing the kinds of pollution found on the site. Since this very conspicuous sovereign act, the executive office has used environmental damage and public recognition of several million citizen-victims of radioactive fallout to emphasize Kazakhstan's staunch opposition to nuclear weapons.[40] Making this once-secret toxic landscape visible was a rallying point for a post-Soviet national identity, but tellingly, in terms of blame, the negative health effects of radiation exposure are confined to the Soviet era.[41] Some two million people in Kazakhstan from 711 settlements received "radiation passports," entitling them to some form of monetary compensation and medical benefits, as well as early retirement.[42] Present-day concerns from local medical doctors and environmental organizations about residual radioactivity in and around the Polygon are portrayed as out of line with economic development and unhealthy "radiophobic" thinking.

I heard a typical example of such thinking from Damira, an environmental activist opposed to the privatization of the Polygon. "It's crazy to think radiation goes away as if by magic! It is not normal for people to live on a nuclear test site and grow food. [The IRSE] think I am illogical, that I suffer from radiophobia. It's absurd!" She went on to explain how promulgating radiophobia is actually incentivized by the plans to privatize the Polygon:

> For the Institute, privatizing the Polygon means there always is a job. They will spend their time making maps: miners will dig, radiation will migrate, they will map it and get paid. Better yet, they will show there is no radiation and get paid even more. For other researchers it's also great: people live there and animals graze on pastures. You can do any studies you want. Look at Koian: three generations of people ingesting radioactive food. This is a perfect opportunity to do a longitudinal study of intergenerational effects.

And indeed, when speaking of people who challenge the Institute about residual radiation at the Polygon, a key industry official told me, "They're just radiophobic." I was told by one of the scientists working at the Institute that "inciting fear of radiation is a political tool that can impede vital economic development in this region." To prove that the test site is safe, the scientific staff of the NNC and IRSE is quick to point out that their own health be taken as proof positive. Hundreds have been working in the area for years and nothing has come of it.

When I asked IRSE officials about radiation and the Polygon, I was told it was safe to go anywhere I wanted to. "I can go to Chagan Lake?" I asked. The product of an underground nuclear blast in 1965, the crater is more than three hundred feet (one hundred metres) deep and thirteen hundred feet (nearly four hundred metres) in diameter. Of particular concern are the very high levels of radioactive hydrogen (tritium) that contaminate the ground water, and hence the plants, in many parts of this region.[43] Although radioactive contamination of the site is uneven, the shores of the lake have readings one hundred or more times above what is considered normal background radiation.[44] During the hottest summer months, some scientists claim to go swimming there, and in the late 1980s the daring Colonel Nikolai Petrushenko (with a Geiger counter in hand) declared the lake safe and plunged into the cold waters with his twelve-year-old son in front of horrified journalists. I was told as well of cavalier locals who strip down to their underwear and jump in, demonstrating their lack of radiophobia. When I asked if it was really safe to go swimming or whether taking a dip was just thrill-seeking practice, my question was answered with a shrug and this advice: "Sure, but I wouldn't stay in the water for too long."

Containing the Damage

From the perspective of environmental activists in Kazakhstan, radiophobia is a "normalization technique"[45] used to control discussions about radioactive pollution such that issues of public health can be deprioritized while free market policies are embraced.[46] Critics see this syndrome that resides in people's heads as a key political and economic strategy employed by the IRSE to explain the safety of the Polygon, as well as the future development plan for the region. These activists see the Institute's claims about the existence of radiophobia as reflecting Kazakhstan's political and economic commitments to "late capitalism,"[47] which can be understood as increasingly organized around a "biopolitics of disposability."[48] A holdover from the Soviet era, this outlook renders some populations invisible and disposable, including most certainly the poor and other marginalized groups living in and around the site. Seen in this light, radiophobia is a form of denialism, an "ideological position whereby one systematically reacts by refusing reality and truth."[49]

In recent years many international critics, including epidemiologists, medical doctors, psychologists, and other science and social science experts, have come to question radiophobia – especially given that Soviet authorities and international organizations embarked on a sustained disinformation campaign and cover-up of the Chornobyl (Chernobyl) accident, withholding necessary information for making health claims.[50] Some critics argue that, in minimizing the health impact of Chornobyl (Chernobyl) and locating it in the minds of victims rather than in the context of radiation exposure itself, radiophobia has become a powerful tool of the nuclear lobby and amounts to a "blame the victim" mentality.[51]

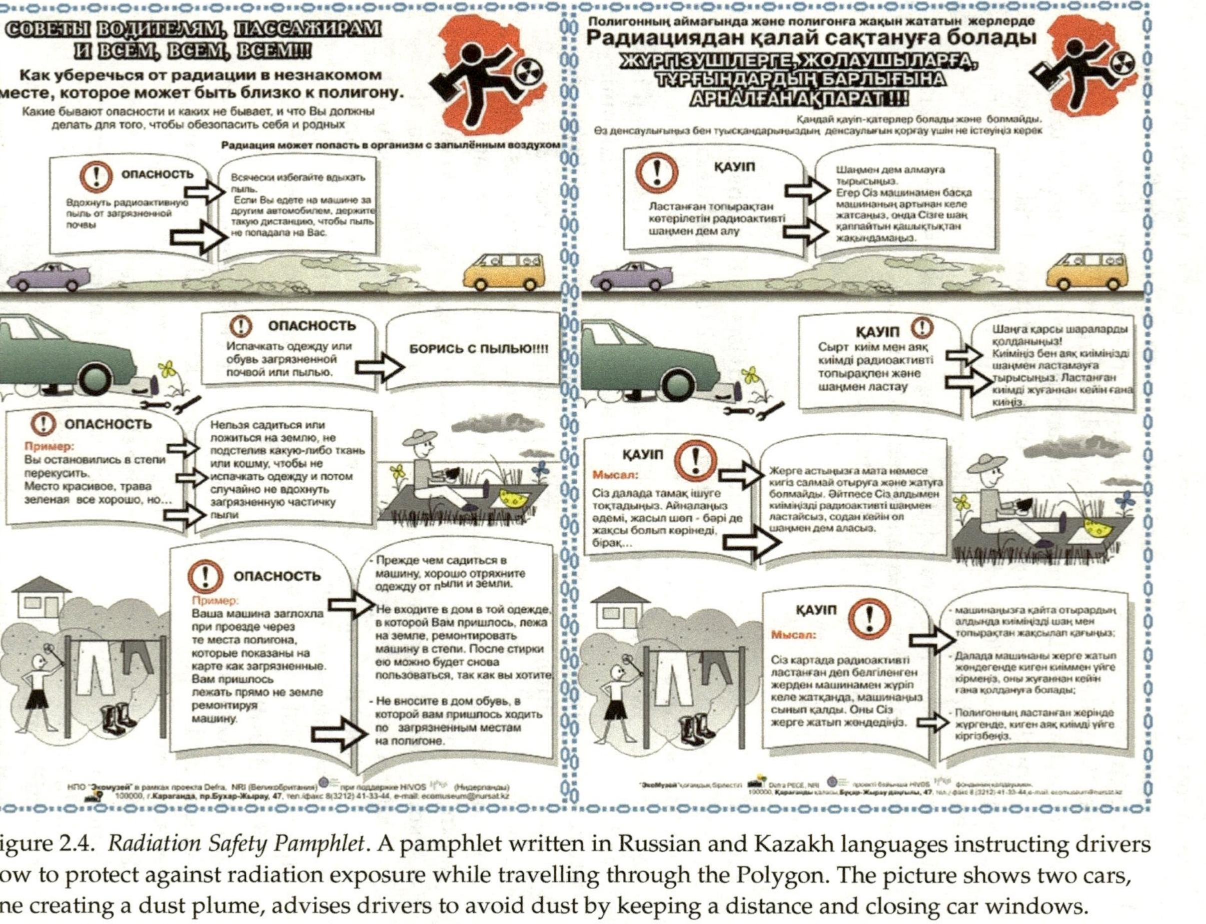

Figure 2.4. *Radiation Safety Pamphlet*. A pamphlet written in Russian and Kazakh languages instructing drivers how to protect against radiation exposure while travelling through the Polygon. The picture shows two cars, one creating a dust plume, advises drivers to avoid dust by keeping a distance and closing car windows. Cartoon illustrations below caution against fixing cars or picnicking on the polluted ground of the test site. The pamphlet also advises people to change clothes used on the test site before entering their homes because of potential dust contamination with residual radioactive elements.

In Kazakhstan matters are quite different – with virtually no exclusion zones relative to the size of the site and economic activity spread across the Polygon, there has been little in the way of studies on psychological health or the impact from residual radiation exposure.[52] The Institute has come to refer mostly to the psychological effects of radiophobia, with little statistical data or peer-reviewed scientific research that would permit quantification of behaviours associated with real or perceived radiation exposure. With little incentive on the part of IRSE to protect the population from potential harms associated with radiation, Semyon's environmental organization developed its own education program to deal with the problem. According to Semyon (an expert in radioecology), the goal of the project was to dissuade individuals living in and around the Polygon from dangerous activities by "helping people to help themselves." Public meetings were organized by environmental organizations using instructive cartoons and theatre plays on radiation safety. Posters in Russian and Kazakh were distributed to residents, including "advice for drivers" on how to safely travel through the Polygon by car.

The environmental organization's minimal intervention was a balancing act between denial and concession, framing radiation as an actual problem with the environment but one that the locals had to navigate on their own.

As another director of a local environmental organization based in Almaty told me, a more realistic appraisal of the Polygon would acknowledge that the focus on nuclear energy production and economic development is meant to deflect discussions of cleaning up the test site – including whether rehabilitation is even possible given that long-lasting radioisotopes like plutonium, with a half-life of over twenty-four thousand years, cannot be contained. Wind, water flow, and soil erosion make it likely (if not inevitable) that the radioisotopes will migrate, and the sheep, goats, cows, and horses grazing on radioactive pastures will be sold in city markets, spreading radioactivity and causing genetic damage.

Local scientists have come to use evidence of genetic mutations in their efforts to draw "more international attention to Semipalatinsk – both in terms of humanitarian aid and further radiobiological investigation of the relationship between radiation and cancer."[53] A key source is the work of Ukrainian geneticist Yuri Dubrova and colleagues,[54] who found that aboveground nuclear tests conducted in Kazakhstan increased genetic "minisatellite mutations" among local populations and that these "junk DNA" mutations are transmitted from parents to offspring. Higher rates of such germ-line mutations were found in children of populations living in and around the Polygon than in the chosen control group. Despite this important finding, Dubrova's team did not associate genetic damage with illness because the study could not link negative health outcomes to genetic mutations, nor could it be replicated among atomic bomb survivors.[55] Nonetheless, some in Kazakhstan's medical establishment interpret Dubrova's findings as evidence that radiation leads to grave consequences in the germ line and in subsequent generations.

Although the link between mutation and congenital abnormalities has yet to be proved, *mutation* has another currency in Kazakhstan – not only as a call for humanitarian aid but also as a way to suggest that residents of the Polygon are biologically corrupt. This has led the country's medical establishment to showcase the Polygon as "proof" that the legacy of nuclear testing is long-term intergenerational genetic damage. In 2012, President Nazarbaev launched Abolish Testing: Our Mission (ATOM), an international campaign aimed at permanently stopping global nuclear testing by highlighting the devastating human effects of radioactive exposure. The message on the campaign's website is potent: "We know that nuclear weapons testing has horrifying consequences. Even today, children are born with severe deformities related to their exposure to nuclear radiation from testing conducted years ago."[56] This view was buttressed by the documentary film *After the Apocalypse*,[57] which features Boris Gusev, a medical doctor and expert in radiobiology, who worked at the Institute of Radiation Medicine and Ecology (formerly the clandestine radiation clinic known as Dispensary No. 4). In the film, Gusev refers to "the children of parents who have been irradiated":

> We thought that everything would go smoothly, that chromosomal damage and genetic effects would be confined only to the generation of people who were irradiated, and they would not be inherited by future generations. But it turned out that this was wrong.

Countless medical doctors, government officials, and NGO workers have come to the same conclusion and see the rural residents of the Polygon as a "genetic underclass" who should be barred from reproducing.[58] Some doctors interviewed in the documentary film and during my own fieldwork went as far as to call for implementing genetic passports that would be used to protect untainted citizens from the so-called mutant stock and thus prevent a "genetic catastrophe."

The Koianer Response

Debates about radiophobia and genetic mutation leave the Polygon populations on the margins of social and political recognition. Seen as victims of the Soviet past, the rural poor are denied any meaningful right of recompense and instead are viewed as "bare life"[59] whose cellular materials and disposable labour are commodified[60] and whose "humanitarian moment" has long since passed.[61] This unravelling is manifested in residents' failure to demand state action and in their denial of how severe the environmental damage is. Koianers don't demand a clean environment because they are "adapted" to their environment. Their political demobilization is further exacerbated by limited access to social welfare and the local emergence of free market capitalism, with science and the market becoming the state's tools for sustaining a resource-based economy centred on producing uranium and oil at the expense of environmental cleanup.

The options presented to the residents of the Polygon seem quite limited: if they express any reservations about radiation, they would be told (by state authorities) their fears are all in their head and they suffer from radiophobia and (by some physicians) that their victimization makes them unacceptable as genetic mutants to be shunned at all costs. But rather than accept these narratives, Koianers and the residents of the Polygon have reworked the debates about low-dose radiation into everyday narratives where they emerged not as victims but as evolutionary advances. Most have come to see themselves as hardened by radiation, genetically adapted and immune to its effects. Among Koianers, illnesses that others might consider symptoms of radiation-related sickness were regarded as a physical manifestation of this adaptation – their emergent mutant subjectivities that provoke particular "modes of perception, affect, thought, desire, [and] fear."[62]

This is not to say that Koianers were healthy. Koianers insisted that years of radiation exposure made everyone "a little sick," as Burkut said, but that they have survived and live long lives. Looking through a list of medical records given to me by a regional nurse, I saw that anaemia, cancer, hypertension, headaches, skin rashes, and bone pain were common. Many had at one point in their lives suffered hair loss, frequent nosebleeds, unexplainable skin burns, and cataracts. For those living with these disabling ailments, they were self-explanatory – the daily effects of low-dose radiation exposure. And it is true that everyone I met in Koian had a family member who died of cancer. But the "severe deformities" described by the medical establishment were

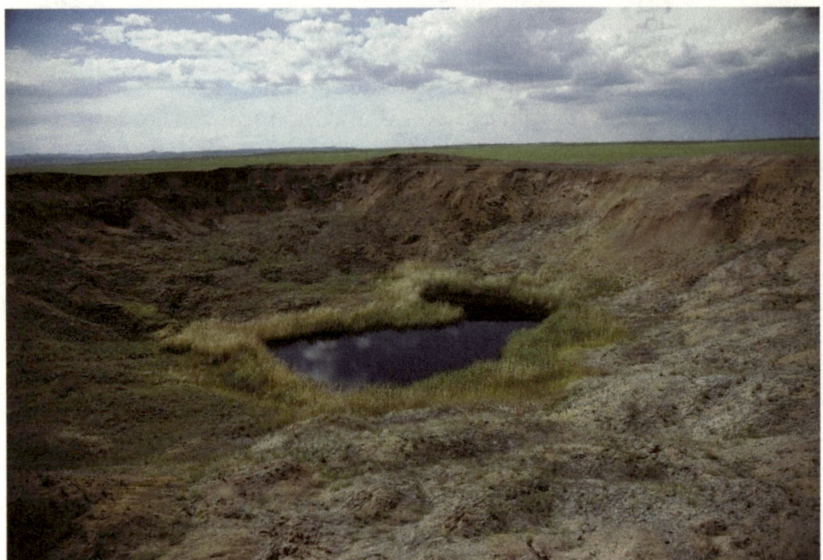

Figure 2.5. *Nuclear Watering Hole*. Nuclear crater formed from underground blast, with a small blue lake now serving as a convenient watering hole for livestock in an area with limited water resources.

simply not present, and they seemingly had avoided becoming the "genetic failures" predicted by the medical establishment.[63]

Yet in Koian, most people considered themselves mutants in the sense of being biologically different from other human populations and from their own ancestors. Although they might not have seen themselves as radioactive, they nevertheless considered themselves the products of radioactive processes. Residents believe something quite different from what anthropologist Adriana Petryna[64] heard from survivors of the Chornobyl (Chernobyl) accident about their ability to tough it out in a toxic environment. And while individual perspectives varied, most believed that their bodies have adapted to a radioactive ecosystem and, like the mutants of atomic age science fiction, consequently thrive in it. In a sense they mirrored Otto Binder's[65] cautionary tale about the consequences of atomic radiation, seeing themselves as superior beings, able to survive in an environment outsiders can't.

Koianers are not the only ones who think adapting to a radioactive ecosystem is possible. Some regional experts have come to the same conclusion. During the summer of 2012, for example, at a conference at the medical university in the city of Karaganda, a biologist angrily asserted that although all Polygon residents suffer from genetic injuries and transmit them to future generations, they are not serious. "If we [Kazakhs] are the people who live on irradiated land, then we have survived – we have adapted. If we are mutants, as you describe, I say we are more than OK! Look at Magda," he said in a booming voice, referring to me. "She lived in and around the Polygon for years now, and she is still fine." Although I did not live on the Polygon for years like Koian residents, he took my presence there and my survival as proof that adaptation is possible. The proof was that the people of Koian are "normal, born without deformities," as he put it.

Proof of adaptation was also "cultivated"[66] by a variety of encounters.[67] Let me give but one example of such an encounter. In September 2008, a group of international researchers and nuclear scientists with the Comprehensive Test Ban Treaty Organization (CTBTO) visited the Polygon to conduct an integrated field exercise (IFE). Designed to simulate an on-site inspection, the IFE is one of the CTBTO's key means of testing a global alarm system designed to detect clandestine nuclear explosions anywhere in the world. This was the first of its kind at the Semipalatinsk Test Site and the largest in CTBTO history. Dubbed the "ultimate verification measure," this particular IFE aimed to be as "realistic a setting as possible."[68] To achieve this, the scientists invented the state of Arcania on the Polygon – a makeshift tent city where the two hundred participants attempted to uncover and record the source of a fictionalized seismic event and an inexplicable release of caesium-137. For identification purposes, the teams of playacting inspectors, member states observers, NGOs, and media representatives wore different-coloured caps, and most donned protective suits and masks to shield against fictionalized radiation exposure. The CTBTO's website describes their journey and temporary encampment as follows:

> Located eight hours away within the former nuclear test area, the trip took them across a country that was virtually uninhabited apart from the occasional cow or horse. Soon after entering the former nuclear test ground, or the Polygon, as it is known in Kazakhstan, the paved road turned into a field track, taking the bus past deserted buildings belonging to the old nuclear test site. On the evening of 3 September, the teams arrived at the Base of Operations which presented itself as a small settlement of about 30 white and green tents dotted across the landscape. Apart from a tiny village in the distance, no other sign of human habitation was visible in the distance of the Kazakh plains.[69]

For nearly six weeks, teams conducted observation flights in a helicopter while others in bodysuits and respirators worked with ground-penetrating radar, wandered around with magnetometers, and gathered soil samples. Moreover, everyone working inside the inspection site perimeter had to undergo radiation-protection procedures that included a full-body scan with a Geiger counter. For this production, fifty tons of equipment was shipped to the remote location.

The "tiny village in the distance" mentioned on the CTBTO website was Koian. When I arrived two years later to start my fieldwork, Koianers were still talking about it and what they saw: imported food and water, men in bodysuits and masks, and people walking around with strange-looking radiation-measuring devices. When asked about the event, Ramazan offered this insightful reflection:

> We don't know what they were doing there. All we know is that radiation must have been high. That's why they had to wear suits and masks. They would obviously die otherwise. This is why they left all of the masks, suits, and other trash behind. We burned it later in our kitchen stoves. Obviously they knew we are adapted. Why else would they not give us protective clothing?

Conclusion

Burkut once told me, "We eat [radiation]. Slowly and quietly, our bodies got used to it." The people of Koian consciously think of themselves as part of an ecosystem, as organisms that have learned to thrive on a polluted landscape. They train their bodies to acquire biological resistance to radiation's deleterious effects by eating gelatin candy and *mumie* (thought to be calcified bat droppings) and drinking *kumys* (mare's milk) and vodka – small antidotes, or "radioprotectors," believed to absorb radioactive particles but leave enough of them for people to adjust.[70]

Vodka, in particular, is frequently recommended by physicians who swear by its antiradiation properties. This is how people in Koian protect themselves from radiation to remain healthy enough to work in the mines and continue living in the Polygon.

It could be argued that when Koianers insist that they have adapted to radiation, they are drawing on a hybrid strain of Lysenkoism. According to this Soviet-era theory of heredity, which rejected Mendelian genetics in favour of Lamarckian evolutionary ideals, acquired characteristics – such as adaptability to radiation, in this case – are passed on to future generations. But the legacy of Lysenkoism cannot fully

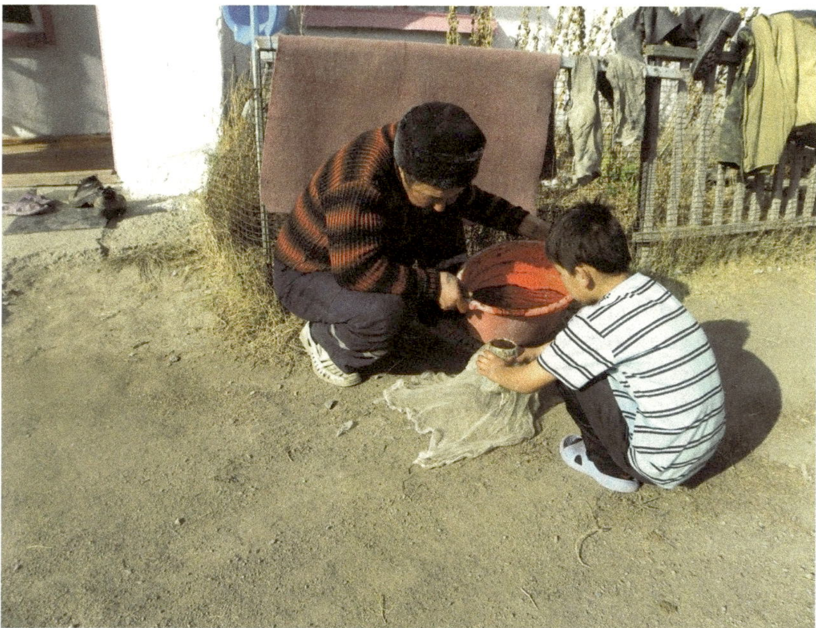

Figure 2.6. *Preparing Traditional Medicine.* A village elder is teaching his grandson how to prepare mumie, a tar-like organic-mineral substance found in the mountain crevices outside of Koian. This collected material, also known as shilajit, has been used as traditional medicine in Central Asia, Russia, China, Pakistan, and elsewhere for thousands of years. In Koian, it is used as treatment for various ailments, including infectious diseases, skin conditions, and respiratory illnesses (like tuberculosis), among others.

account for how people have come to accept their irradiated biology as genetically evolved and perfectly suited to their ecosystem. This is a much more recent and complex phenomenon. After all, most people in Koian and elsewhere in the region learned of radiation-induced genetic damage and mutations only after the Soviet Union collapsed.

Their reconceptualizing of the biological self could instead reflect Kazakhstan's drive to establish itself as a global leader in uranium mining while asserting itself as a victim of the Soviet-era militarization on which it stakes its sovereignty. In this view, the reconceptualized biological self that lives in and around the Polygon captures the future and past of Kazakhstan's nation-building narrative, as well as its position in the global political economy. It also captures the uncertainties in scientific circles about the biological effects of low-dose radiation and the evidence that some organisms have indeed adapted to radioactive environmental conditions.[71] Memories of nuclear testing and contested ways of knowing how irradiated genes shape human biology have allowed them to generate "new understandings of self, nature, and society."[72]

While the conviction held by those living in the region – that they are biologically adapted to radiation – may seem paradoxical, it is a perfectly reasonable response under the circumstances. Because they are left to deal with environmental problems on their own, their only option is to become (or believe themselves to be) enhanced human beings who can survive in toxic environments. To adapt is, moreover, to retain a sense of dignity and agency while surviving in a harsh post-Soviet economic climate. By saying that they are used to radiation, Koianers avoid engaging with a medical establishment that sees them as biologically damaged victims, with an economic system that offers them very little, and with a judgmental population that sees them as genetically corrupted and rejects their rural and, in many ways, still very collective way of life. In other words, Koianers orient themselves away from mainstream society, refusing to be tied down by a set of scientific categories in a world of limited economic opportunities or strategies for happiness.[73] In sum, they embody a global "mutant ecology"[74] that has transformed their very view of life.

3 "Sami Po Sebe": Economy on the Periphery

The camp doesn't need successive cataclysms or bombs raining down on its inhabitants to enjoy mutual aid and fatalistic brotherhood.

– Antoine Volodine, Radiant Terminus

Introduction

The winter before I arrived, the pastures around Koian's radioactive landscape froze solid. As temperatures held steady at minus forty degrees Fahrenheit (minus forty degrees Celsius), the animals were unable to punch through the thick sheet of ice. "Cows don't dig with their hooves; they use their heads," Tursynbek said. For months, everyone in the village tried uncovering the grassy fields with shovels. It wasn't long before the cows began to starve. By winter's end, some one hundred animals died – almost the entire herds belonging to two families – transforming the ice-covered fields into their macabre resting place. With the arrival of spring's warm temperatures, the entire village began to smell with the intensity of the decomposing corpses that were now also black with millions of flies. "The stench was horrible," Tursynbek's wife Altynai shared. "For weeks, everything – our clothes, houses, air – reeked of rotting flesh. We had to deal with this situation quickly." Before the animals sank into the knee-deep mud with the spring rains, the residents of Koian hauled them over the hill to a garbage pile and set fire to them.

When I first arrived at Koian, people were still reeling from this catastrophic *koshmar* (nightmare). This devastating winter not only had decimated animal herds but had left the residents struggling for survival on a daily basis. I was told that by February the village had little food left and in springtime everyone's clothing had grown considerably baggier.

But going hungry was only part of the challenges they faced that year. Coal supplies were dwindling by mid-winter and no one was able to keep their homes warm. There was no help from the *akim* (mayor) in Oktiabr' either. The frequent *burany* (blizzards) and the drifting, deep snow made walking to the town for supplies impossible. Koian was essentially cut off from the rest of the world for four months.

Harbouring the memories of the previous year, everyone in the village during the September of my arrival was busy preparing, fearing the worst. They were gathering extra hay, purchasing additional coal from a nearby mine, and buying various food products in bulk at the Karaganda city *bazar* (market). Some of the men managed to pick up extra shifts at the open pit mine on the Polygon. However, most residents lacked the money to buy everything necessary and ended up bartering for goods, borrowing cash from relatives, or purchasing items on *kredit* (credit) at a tiny family-run store in Oktiabr'.

When I returned to Koian in the summer of 2012, things in the village had not improved. The steppe roads, already barely passable on the driest of days, were even more rutted and difficult to traverse. Koian's primary grade school was permanently closed and so was its one-room medical clinic. The village was without power for nearly a month because one of the poles connecting Koian to Oktiabr' had overturned during a storm, and the administrators of Oktiabr' refused to fix the problem, "exhausted" by helping people who choose to live in "primitive conditions." Perhaps the most significant setback was when the boss of the local Polygon mine fired nearly all the area employees for several months. Those let go were offered an alternative: to work in a mine located some seven hundred miles (more than one thousand kilometres) away for significantly lower pay. The company "graciously" offered transportation from Oktiabr', and without much of a choice, many agreed to go.

The horror stories of animal deaths and the tales of starvation and depravation were told again and again. But what surprised me the most was the fact that these many trials didn't impact people's choice to stay in Koian. The akim has been begging villagers for years to move to Oktiabr' and even offered them housing and access to animal pastures. But Koianers refused to abandon their village and claimed the akim was trying to make their lives harder on purpose to get them to move. "How else do you explain why the akim didn't plow the steppe road when we were stuck for months?" Tursynbek said. Like the other villagers, he often would say how they preferred to live *sami po sebe* (on their own and keeping to themselves) rather than move and "pay for houses and pastures with no access to natural watering places that would only further line the pockets of the lazy and money-hungry local administrators who could care less about them."[1]

In Koian, sami po sebe captures a wealth of different meanings and feelings about people's lives as they experience them. It can mean that Koianers are forced to fend for themselves, abandoned by the state and local administrators. But it also speaks very directly to how they struggle through days and seasons to maintain their rural home and livelihoods on their own, where they are free of economic pressures associated with urban life or those that people face in Oktiabr'. Although everyone knows that it's much harder and uncomfortable to live in Koian, life is more fraternal than the one embodied and experienced outside it.[2] Sami po sebe is the narrative context, the setting, and the actions through which Koianers have reinvented a cooperative enterprise for themselves – a kind of "neosocialist corporation," or an atomic collective, where everyday life is not dictated by maximizing profits, but rather by the concern for collective survival of the village through mutual assistance.[3] Their precariousness "implies living socially," depending on networks of support.[4] It's a survival strategy antithetical to market-driven life and a response to unequal wealth production and distribution of resources beyond the village after the fall of the Soviet Union.

What I learned is that sami po sebe allows Koianers to live mostly apart from an economic order that has no room for them and privileges the near-universal ideal of holding down a "proper [salaried] job."[5] They have embraced what cultural historian Michael Denning[6] has called "wageless life": a collective existence as subsistence livestock breeders at the margins of the marketplace where they have (at least in principle) co-operative control over the means to "survive and thrive beyond waged labor."[7] In Koian, sami po sebe is more than a situation marked by extreme scarcity and marginality, or lives that scholars have often framed as "precarious," "bare," and "marginal" – where subsistence livestock breeding is the "last resort" for the unemployed trying to survive in extreme poverty.[8] Yet none of these terms adequately capture how Koianers live or what they desire. Tursynbek and others insist that despite everything, theirs is a "good life," and no one in Koian "lives in poverty." To understand why people prefer to survive on livestock breeding on the Polygon rather than find waged employment elsewhere, we must understand how villagers have given new meaning and purpose to their lives through subsistence labour, or as anthropologist Kathleen Millar aptly states, "how life becomes livable through forms of labour commonly defined in terms of redundancy, abandonment, or exhaust."[9]

What exactly does it mean for villagers to be part of Koian's livestock breeding collective after the sovkhoz collapsed? How is labour organized? What are the conduits of their economic existence? How are their broader goals built into their efforts? Their isolation and reinvention into a collective farm have come to form the very basis of their solidarity: how they actually subsist, build relationships, make meaning, and reproduce their collective existence. But theirs is also a complex and inherently flexible system that to be understood required me to follow people's movements in the context of their geography and economics as well as the tight labour and organizational structure, which simultaneously provides a sense of meaning and order for their collective enterprise.

Envisioning the Collective

The economic pressures brought on by Kazakhstan's switch to market capitalism in the 1990s meant that salaried jobs in places like Koian, which were plentiful during the Soviet era, became virtually non-existent. This is perhaps surprising given that international organizations that monitor the economic, political, and social progress of so-called "developing" nations consistently celebrate Kazakhstan as Central Asia's miracle – a state clearly on the path to meet all eight United Nations Millennium Development Goals.[10] Its success has much to do with its export-oriented resource-based economy, especially oil.[11] Reports from the World Bank are filled with positive assessments for the country – its "impressive reduction in poverty," "commendable progress" in managing the environmental impact of industries, and its ability to transform the command economy to one dictated by privatization as defined in the "ease of doing business" rankings.[12]

But these reports highlight only a part of the story. State actors in Kazakhstan had little choice but to reconfigure the economic system along neoliberal lines, including the liquidation of previously state-controlled enterprises and the overhaul of state protections that formerly served a rationalized welfare program.[13] Western advisers, researchers, and multinational corporations drove the terms of the "shock therapy" – the rapid conversion to free market economics and policy making that favour private enterprise and limited government regulation – and in the process created the conditions where wealth became concentrated in Kazakhstan's new governing elites, while people like those living in Koian were dispossessed of their property, work, and social protections, and divested of their social status.[14] The neoliberal shifts also affected healthcare. State funding was drastically reduced, eliminating the position of the village doctor, and the trend towards privatization resulted in a new two-tier system in which public healthcare was maintained to a limited extent while paid care expanded, leaving many individuals with no or limited access to doctors and medicine.

Meanwhile, Kazakhstan offered its cheap natural resources, human labour, and other commodity markets to enthusiastic venture capitalists and multinational banks and corporations ready to compete for scarce economic and political resources of the formerly isolated market space.[15] Some of the world's largest global multinationals directly invest in Kazakhstan, which has semi-privatized its extraction economy.[16] These include ArcelorMittal, the second-biggest steel producer in the world with mines and steel plants operating in Karaganda and Temirtau, Canada's Cameco, and Kazakhstan's own Kazatomprom, a major supplier of nuclear fuel services. The tangled international web woven by neoliberalism is neatly illustrated by the Tengizchevroil company – a joint venture between Chevron; ExxonMobil; the Russian, US, and British LukArco; and Kazakhstan's KazMunayGas – which has a majority stake in the exploration and development of the Tengiz oil field.[17]

For Koianers, the economic restructuring programs didn't translate to a better standard of living. It mostly meant that people lost jobs while subsidies for education, healthcare, and infrastructure could no longer be counted on. It's no wonder the countless World Bank development graphs, statistics, and future projections about the positive economic development of the country are irrelevant in the day-to-day lives of villagers like those living in Koian. Among the rural poor, there is a refined awareness of the differences between political rhetoric and reality. But while villagers might find themselves holding the "short end of the neoliberal stick"[18] and trapped in what some scholars would see as a dystopian new world order, Koianers don't see themselves only in that way. Their "system" of sami po sebe resides both within and outside the mainstream economy which international observers miss. The various labours and structures that compose Koian's economic activity are based upon a complex infrastructure of knowledge, connections, and participation. How that system fits in with Kazakhstan's broader post-Soviet trajectory is worth remarking upon, if only for the sole reason that it would appear to be a glaring aberration to the story commonly told by the champions of neoliberalism.

When the Soviet Union collapsed, the farm sector, like the rest of the economy, experienced a difficult conversion from a planned to a market economy. As a result, throughout the 1990s, the general state-level policy towards the agricultural sector (including livestock breeding) was mostly that of defunding and neglect.[19] Even though people tried to maintain the former large-scale farms, because Kazakhstan's economy was integrated into the broader economy of the Soviet Union, the collapse caused a significant disruption in the flow of goods, and the high cost of everything made doing so impossible.[20] Although the 1995 Land Code broke up state farms and eventually allowed people to lease parcels from the state for forty-nine-year terms, the sovkhoz went bankrupt.[21] Tursynbek vividly described the end of the sovkhoz approach: "We couldn't buy anything. Even if we could, the prices were too high. We tried to make the farm work like the old sovkhoz for a couple of years, that's what we knew to do, but there was no infrastructure to keep it going."

By the mid-1990s, large-scale livestock farming in Kazakhstan had virtually disappeared, and animals were increasingly concentrated in households for individual consumption.[22] Cash was hard to come by. "All my savings turned to zero. And we got zero support from the state," Tursynbek offered. "So we collected metal instead." When the Polygon was officially closed in 1991 and the army disbanded, the test site was a landscape littered with millions of tons of scrap. With it no longer a military zone (though still contaminated with residual radioactivity), Koianers scavenged the site during those turbulent early years of independence for whatever they could find and dismantled any infrastructure left over. Stories told around the table recount how people dug pipes and cables out of the ground with picks and shovels, carting carloads of material away to the Karaganda bazar. The brief market that emerged for this trade had by the mid-2000s mostly disappeared as most things had already been hauled off. Seasonal grass fires expose stray findings here and there, but only one person in Koian still searches for metal out on the Polygon steppe.

Consistent access to land has remained a central concern. In 2003, the government amended the Land Code to allow for private ownership of agricultural plots.[23] However, this new program is neither a simple nor clear-cut system that enables people to secure land rights, as much of what remains resides under state ownership and is doled out through leases approved by a local akim.[24] No one in Koian has purchased any acreage because Koianers claim the akim only "sells land to the highest bidder – the *latifundists* [large landowners] who keep workers in conditions similar to *rabstvo* [slavery]."[25] In fact, only one villager even leases pastures because the registration process is too costly and burdensome.[26] Instead, the pastures around the village remain communal, including areas of the Polygon that people use. Villagers only lease small areas around their homes, which include barns, water wells, and hay meadows.[27]

On a crisp fall afternoon in 2015, I stopped by the Akimat (town hall) in Oktiabr' in the hopes of studying a map of the sovkhoz to get a better sense of how the area was laid out before the collapse of the Soviet Union compared to how people use the space today. The akim offered me a cup of tea with chocolates and began casually complaining of the stubbornness of Koianers persisting in the village so far out. "I've wished for years for them to move out of there, but they just refuse. And we're an extended family! They should relocate to Oktiabr', so I don't have to worry about them overturning the tractor or getting them out of the mud," the akim said. We then turned to other local events like power outages.

After a mandatory gossip session, the akim led me to an office where a large, faded map hung on a dark paneled wall – actually an agronomic chart designed by the Kazakhstan Institute for Land Planning (Kazgiprozem) in 1982 that depicted Oktiabr' and the territories under its jurisdiction. Heavily weathered, it had been used by state economists in the field whose job was to make the landscape ordered and productive. But it was also a window into how Soviet cartographers recorded reality as they saw it. In colourful layers of elaborate topographic detail, they drew bands of green, blue, pink, yellow, and orange as pastures, meadows, wetlands, lakes, and arable fields spreading outward from Oktiabr' and towards the hills. Over colour-shaded areas, they drew inky shapes and delicate lines that mingled with hard-edged contours, half-circles, and crosses as they plotted settlements and the specific characteristics of vegetation, soil, and water quality. The layers turned the map into a two-dimensional nesting doll: one large field divided into smaller and smaller sections, each assigned a number and a purpose, connected as one. On top of the map were three wind rose diagrams depicting the general direction of wind patterns (southwest) for the fall and spring, as well as the entire year.

Hanging on the wall, the map is a historical artefact that provides a throughline of the area's agricultural history while also giving a sense of continuity to a political and economic system that has largely been reimagined. Soviet mapmakers saw this landscape as a vast economic resource and went to great efforts to chart the region in exact and specific terms. For the agronomists, it was a kind of thick topographic description for ordering space, easy to envision people sowing fields, vast combines unloading grain at collection stations, and flocks of sheep waiting for a shearing. Like all maps, this one offered a particular perspective.

Today, most of this activity has ceased, and only livestock breeding remains. It is now a dominant source of income for all households, but unlike during the Soviet era, the animals are primarily raised for subsistence (non-cash income) to supplement the meagre wages people get from pensions and other piecemeal work.

But the activity also represents a rejection of the market economy that has come to dominate Kazakhstan after the fall of the Soviet Union in favour of envisioning the endeavour as a collective effort. Family

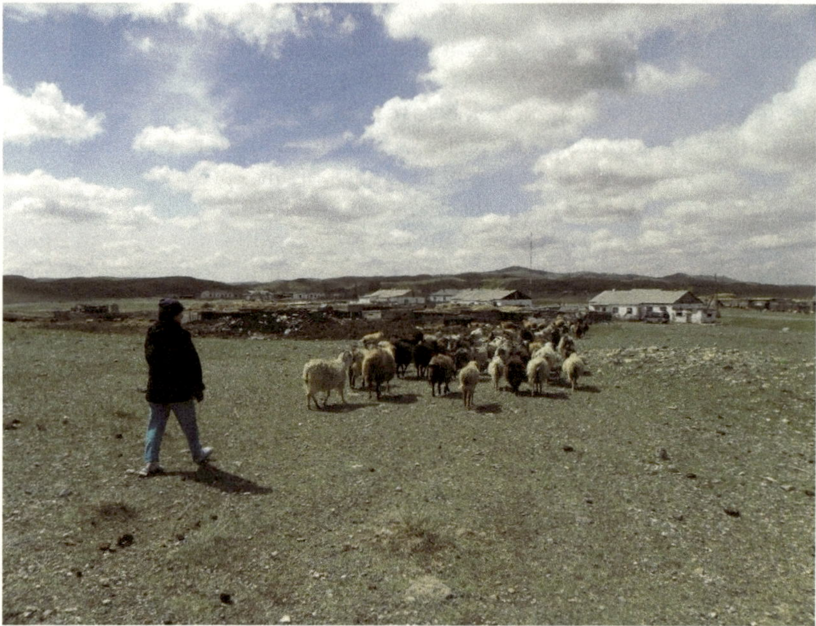

Figure 3.1. *Bringing in the Flock.* A woman bringing sheep in from the pastures at the end of the day. Today, men tend to the sheep during the day in the fields several kilometres away from Koian, while women help guide them back to the barn in the evening.

resources are pooled into a system in which networking (often based on reciprocal favours or *blat*) as well as gift giving and social and kinship ties provide stability amidst limited resources.[28] Everyone is expected to contribute to Koian's overall well-being, and all help is returned in kind. In case of an emergency, like the winter livestock die off or seasonal steppe fires, everyone comes together to share resources. The same goes for finding missing livestock (or searching for a thief) in what to anyone outside the village is a vast landscape without reference points.

Although today the fields grow wild, Koianers follow a practice from the Soviet times that their parents and grandparents knew well. Through the movements, habits, and stories of their elders, the younger villagers have acquired a depth of knowledge that includes finding the best fodder, as well as exercising care to rotate where they work to avoid over-harvesting. Hay is collected at the end of every summer and into early fall to feed the livestock through the long winters. They work

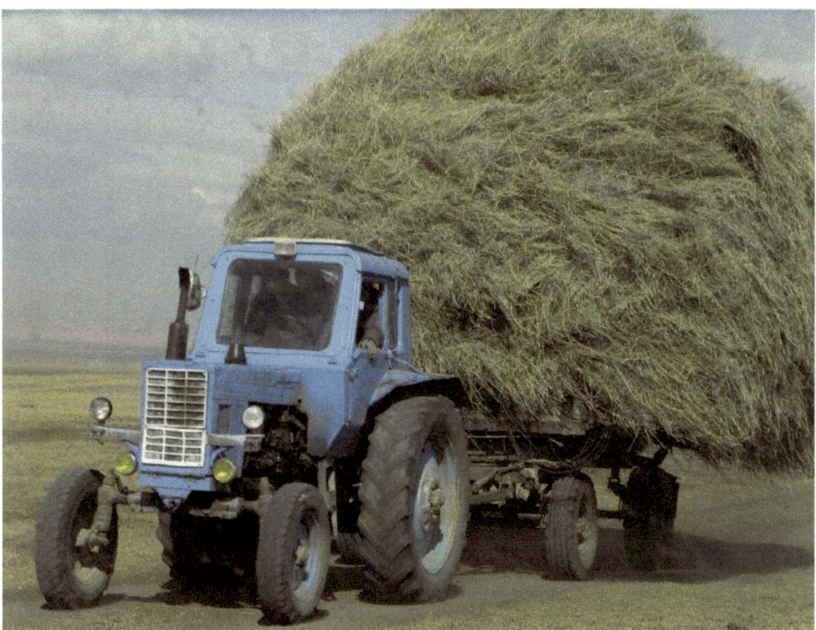

Figure 3.2. *Hay Collecting*. The hay was gathered in the fields outside the village and will be stacked high on the roofs of barns upon returning to Koian.

what are now the abandoned Virgin Lands agricultural fields – some ten miles (sixteen kilometres) from the village, just beyond a rugged mountain ridge and along a makeshift dirt road. Backs bent under the weight of dried straw, they use broken pitchforks to throw it high onto a wagon pulled by their powder blue tractor that Ramazan owns, but the village collectively uses and maintains. The mosquitoes and biting flies incessantly gnaw at their bodies.

While I was in Koian, I was asked to shuttle lunches of tea and dried mutton with deep-fried biscuits to those working under the blazing sun. Despite the scorching temperatures and backbreaking work, they talk and laugh, surrounded by the quiet grasslands in a seemingly desolate landscape. But their work is not done. House by house, climbing upon every barn, they chuck the straw onto the flat rooftops well into the night. Over time the mounting piles of hay give the village its winter look. This annual routine usually takes five to eight weeks of cutting, stacking, loading, transporting, and piling these much-prized fodder crops until there's enough to last their animals through the long winter.

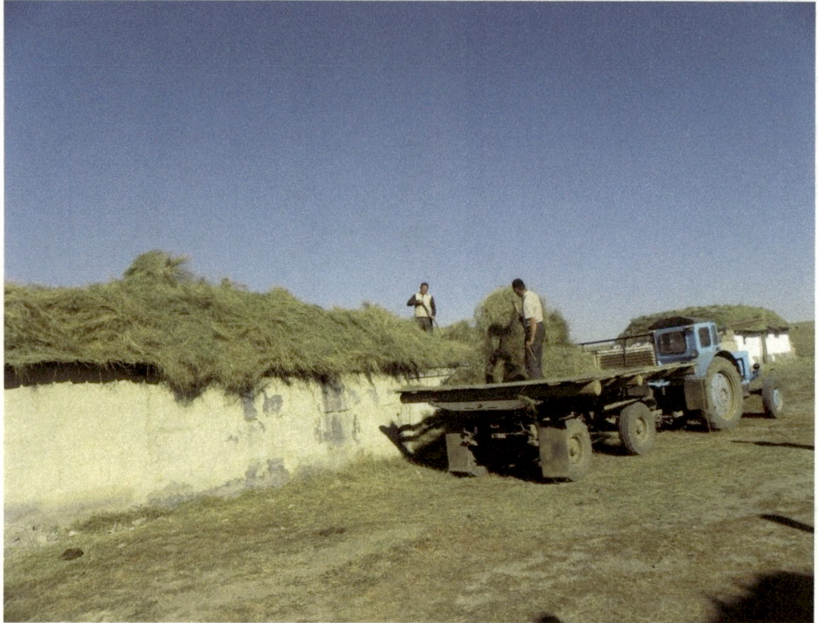

Figure 3.3. *Piling Hay on Barn Rooftops*. Men using pitchforks to unload hay onto a barn roof in early fall. This hay will feed livestock through the winter.

Considering the map in the akim's office, life in the village is truly between worlds. By reinventing their collective farm after the fall of the Soviet Union, the village has become the lynch pin of a broader (yet ironic) strategy of upward mobility – ironic because Koianers remain both within and independent of discourses about "informal economies," "precarity," and "insecurity."[29] How they live shows a deepening of social support networks – what others have called an "informal economy" to make life near abandoned nuclear landscape a more desirable alternative than to move away – or in the words of Tursynbek, "at least we had milk and eventually meat when the herds got bigger."[30]

Trip to the Bazar

One summer morning in 2012, Tursynbek and four other village men got up at dawn – when the temperatures were still cool – to slaughter a cow. They woke me as well, anxious not to get a late start as summer temperatures and the eight-hour journey to the winding rows, stalls, and back alleys of the bazar in Karaganda would spoil the meat.[31] This day a sheep was also slaughtered; this would go to Tursynbek and Altynai's three older children who live in the city. The combined load – about 150 kilograms, or 330 pounds – was neatly wrapped in a large blue tarp and placed in the back of my Delica van.

Before departing, I asked if anyone in the village needed a ride to Oktiabr' or needed anything else along the way. Grocery orders were plenty: I gathered itemized lists of *produkty* (typically referring to food, but in Koian produkty could also mean any household merchandise, like detergents, hair colouring solutions, or medicine). That day the orders included about three hundred pounds (about 130 kilograms) of flour, sugar, and rice; three large sacks of carrots and onions; twenty boxes of black tea; ten heads of cabbage; four large buckets of lime for painting houses; and a much-awaited electric *separator* (a machine that divides milk into cream and skimmed milk, from which butter, sour milk, yogurt, and *qurt* – dried sour skimmed milk – are made). Because the price of produkty is at least four times cheaper in the city than in the small and often inadequately stocked family-run store in Oktiabr', people always buy merchandise in bulk.

On this particular day, I received an education in what it means to navigate the workings of Koian's rural economy and piecemeal wage labour vis-à-vis the city. Tursynbek and Altynai usually joined me on trips to the city – in part to make sure that their village commodities arrived safely to their destination and in part to visit with their other children. This time, however, they stayed behind. I was not returning immediately, and without a reliable car (which no one in the village had at the time), it would be difficult for them to piece together a way back to Koian using buses, taxis, and other inconveniences that could take days. Tursynbek was also about to begin his monthly two-week shift at a nearby mine working twelve hours a day, so there was no time for him to take a trip.

The isolation of Koian, lack of transportation, and bad weather conditions mean that villagers encounter considerable difficulties in selling livestock. Of course, selling anything was prohibited during the Soviet times and the term *kommersant* (businessperson, seller, or trader) captured a great deal of the moral and ethical problems associated with this economic activity, carrying with it the same negativity and accusation from the Soviet era. Saying someone is a kommersant means that they are morally suspect because they own a business only to "make money for themselves" through sheer exploitation, and they are by default a thief. The small home-based storeowners in Oktiabr' or people who charge money for shuttling animals to market are consistently critiqued for price gouging and for trying to get rich without considering other peoples' economic circumstances.[32] Those who barter, sell livestock, or other goods to support their family or the village are not considered to be kommersanty, and even selling is a relatively new phenomenon in Koian, dating back only to the fall of the sovkhoz. Before then, people relied on the *stepnye biznesmeny* (steppe businessmen) who picked up animals directly from Koian, but today this activity is on the decline and Koianers are obliged to travel long distances and manoeuvre among corrupt buyers, state officials, and local police in the process.

Technically, one can't just take meat from a village and sell it in a city market. There are official steps one must take. For example, all animals must be vaccinated and registered with a local veterinarian. The most important step that the family entrusted me with on this journey was in getting the *spravka* (an official document certifying the meat passed a health inspection and can be transported). During a quick inspection by a livestock vet in another village of the cow's liver for signs of illness, it was determined that the meat was not stolen and that it was also brucellosis and anthrax free and therefore "perfectly fit to eat" (from what I saw there was no scientific evidence to support how this determination was made).[33] The meat they sold (and consumed at home) was not checked for radiation. There were not any tools to measure such a thing, nor were there any state safeguards in place.[34] "We don't know anything about radiation or what is in our food. No one tells us anything," Tursynbek said.

After seven hours of driving, I arrived on the outskirts of Karaganda to collect Tursynbek and Altynai's older son (as well as their nephew and his wife visiting from Koian) from one of the many *khrushchëvki* (concrete five-storey apartment blocks) that dot the outskirts of the city. The son was the one who would actually sell the cow. He was among those family members of Koianers who end up moving away to cities in search of salaried work or education and property ownership. An hour later, with everyone piled inside, we finally reached the back alleys of the bazar and the seemingly random assortment of metal doors enclosing various shops. It was another hour before the kommersant arrived, collected the meat from the van, weighed it, and rolled it into a cooler. The cow's liver was spread out on a large, bloody wooden stump and inspected again for traces of disease. The kommersant – who was an acquaintance of a family friend – didn't bother to look at the spravka, and I only later learned it was really just for the local police in case we were stopped at a random checkpoint. He agreed to buy the entire cow for 135,900 Tenge (USD 924) – not a bad price according to Tursynbek.[35]

I had made this trip on countless occasions, bouncing down the road away from the village, sometimes with a live sheep bound in a potato sack with only its head sticking out.

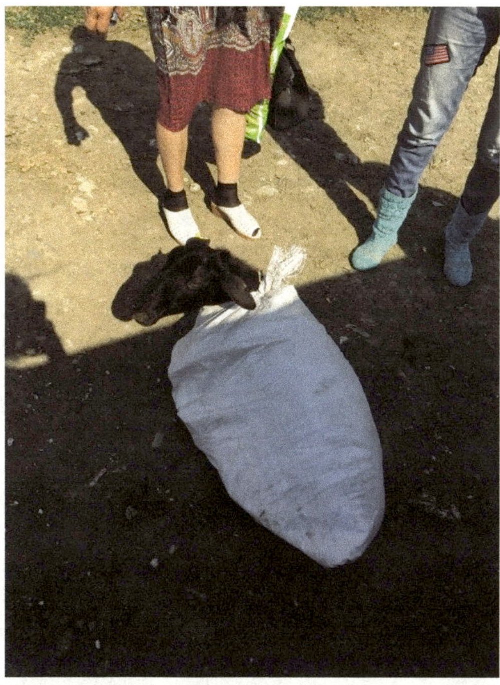

Figure 3.4. *Sheep in a Potato Sack.* This sheep will be taken alive to the market, where it will be sold to a merchant, then slaughtered and sold as meat.

My time and labour were payment of sorts for living in the village. There are transport services that will come to Oktiabr' to pick up meat for delivery, but that adds an additional set of hands for the transaction to go through. The standard cost of carting an animal from Koian to the bazar in Karaganda can be as high as 15,000 Tenge (or USD 102 in 2011)[36] – the equivalent of a month's retirement pension for some or the cost of buying a sheep in 2012.[37]

Part of the money from the sale at the bazar was used to buy produkty for Tursynbek and Altynai's household back in Koian. The rest went to their children in the city who needed help covering food, transportation, and housing costs (in the summer of 2012, it would have been difficult to find a one-room apartment in the city of Karaganda for less than 30,000 Tenge (USD 200) per month – utilities, of course, being extra). Although all of them worked, none had jobs that paid enough to make them fully independent. Like most individuals who moved from

Koian to Karaganda, most rely on their village kin network for financial support, and families pool resources. But because villagers can't sell more than two cows per year without seriously depleting their own food supply, most of the help comes from home-based dairy products such as milk and butter and the occasional meat from a slaughtered sheep – these being more numerous, easier to breed, and much easier to store than cows.[38]

A trip to the bazar provides a snapshot into one aspect of the economy in Koian, showing the linkages between the village and urban areas, as well as illustrating how cash can be made from the collective livestock. But cash isn't the only medium of exchange in Koian that matters on a day-to-day basis. There is actually very little disposable income circulating in the village and barter has mostly replaced monetary exchange, particularly between village residents and those who visit. One could barter several litres of diesel for a ride to Oktiabr' or trade a sheep or two for a couch, rugs, kitchen cabinets, television stands, clothing, and even electronics sold by stepnye biznesmeny. These itinerant traders travelled from one remote village to the next during summer months selling goods from the back of a Kamaz truck. Animals could also be swapped for sets of tires, wheel barrels, and various other types of machinery. Perhaps not surprisingly, Koianers frequently referred to their livestock as a living and breathing "collective bank." While Kazakhstan's government honours Soviet-era pensions, the monthly take-home pay in Koian in 2012 was 16,000 Tenge or approximately USD 110. With the unreliability of the mail service to rural areas and the impassibility of roads in the winter and spring months, these hardly sufficient government funds often arrived late.

How the collective economy functions in terms of its division of labour and movement within the village and beyond brings into sharp relief how group-oriented people's efforts are in contrast to Kazakhstan in a wider sense. Many Koianers remarked on their surroundings – their "ruined life" as they call it both literally and figuratively – noting that the aesthetic is *posle voiny* (after the war). "I was in the military. I went to Moscow, the Czech Republic – I travelled. Many of us did. Now we live like traditional Kazakhs who keep the youngest son in the village and send most of our other children away to the city," Tursynbek said. Yet individuals who moved away to the cities in search of better work found only urban slums on the periphery of cities while remaining chronically unemployed and barely scraping by. Worst of all from the villagers' point of view are the city's psychological effects. As Altynai put it, "I hate being in the city. I'm bored, there's nothing to do. On top of that, I'm alone with my thoughts. Who wants to be alone with their mind?" Koianers reject city life on multiple planes in favour of the village, which represents a life worth living, even if it's characteristically ordered and "traditional."

The Return of Tradition

The collapse of communism had a different effect on women then it did on men. Perhaps one of the defining attributes of the Soviet system was to overcome "tradition" and patriarchal ideologies across its territories, but especially among the Indigenous populations the regime saw as "primitive."[39] The Soviet Union was the first country to enshrine the full liberation of women in its constitution and promoted gender equality across all spheres of life.[40] Although women's advancement was prominent in education, employment, and other spheres of life, they still held secondary roles in government leadership. Women certainly benefited from education and entry into the labour force but nevertheless continued to be saddled with the "double burden" of domestic unpaid work.[41] Culturally and economically speaking, women did experience degrees of professionalization and upward mobility in that system, even if it still was a patriarchal regime. The unravelling of the Soviet Union led to the "Kazakhification" of public life, and with it the "re-traditionalization" of gender roles across post-Soviet space.[42] In Kazakhstan, hierarchized gender relations shifted towards patriarchy and became part of a new nation-building project equating national values with a return to tradition and the so-called "traditional families."[43] The domestic sphere was ascribed to women, while the public one was assigned to men.

In Koian, the dismantling of the sovkhoz economic structure, market-driven poverty, and the revival of patriarchy in Kazakhstan meant that Koianers' duties to the broader collective were transformed along gender lines.[44] For women, this meant their authority and decision-making power became subordinate to that of men. "We used to have real jobs and did everything the men did. We travelled. We were modern. Now we are at home, cooking, cleaning, taking care of the children. We are now living a traditional life," Altynai said. But then she added an illuminating coda: "But without us and our work, Koian can't exist, and I can't imagine myself living in the city for good. What would I do there? I would be bored and just get fat and be alone thinking all the time. I want to be busy." The sense of social, economic, and political dislocation that Altynai describes shows how people were forced to adjust to a new life that (for many) mirrors a forgotten "traditional" Kazakh past.[45] For Altynai, the shift meant a return to domestic work in which housework in the reproduction of life is at once necessary and seen as desirable (compared to the alternative) for sustaining the village collective.[46]

Aigul was born in Oktiabr' and is the daughter of Tursynbek's oldest brother (there were eleven brothers and sisters in total). At the time of my interview, she was thirty-five years old and the mother of two children. Her story, like that of many women, reflects the jarring shift she experienced in terms of gendered expectations compounded by the rural-urban divide. But it also reflects how she has come to see staying in Koian as a much better alternative than leaving:

> I was born near Koian and have family all over. My parents eventually moved to Ekibastuz and I would visit my grandmother in Koian during summer months. She used to be a *banya* [bathhouse] attendant here in Koian. I was a city girl and loved the urban environment. I graduated from high school and became a teacher of Kazakh language. I loved my job. I never imagined I would return to Koian for good. But my father-in-law and his brother arranged for me to be stolen to marry my husband. I was twenty-three years old. It's a tradition, kind of. Many girls are kidnapped in Kazakhstan by men who they then marry. This happens in villages mostly. Sometimes this is arranged by the couple. But I didn't know anything. They just threw me in the car and took me to my now husband's extended family home in Koian to convince me to marry him. I resisted for a whole two days. But I eventually agreed to the marriage because everyone was pressuring me – my friends, his parents, and mine too. The wedding was two weeks later and I remember we drove through ground zero on the Polygon to Semey to take wedding pictures. I never imagined that this would happen to me because I was a city girl.

Since Kazakhstan's independence, the practice of bride abduction has increased. It's a form of marriage practice that exists in many regions of the world, typically involving a man and his friends essentially planning a "kidnapping." It often includes trickery, deception, and physical force to relocate a woman from one place to another with an underlying cultural assumption that she is to become the man's wife.[47] There are numerous versions of this custom and specifics differ in each scenario, such as whether the couple is acquainted, who participates, and the resulting consequences. Many women consent to the union to avoid dishonoring themselves and their families by going against it.[48] The groom's family compensates the bride's family with gifts (horses, sheep, jewellery, or other things), thus establishing new kinship networks.[49] Although all the wives in Koian were abducted, all also knew of their husband's plan ahead of time, effectively making the abduction arranged. Only Aigul's abduction was non-consensual as she did not know ahead of time of her future husband's plans.

Despite the harrowing description of her abduction, Aigul was quick to add this revealing rejoinder to her tale:

> My father-in-law did everything, everything, everything [for me]. He *polnost'iu sdelal menia* [completely made me]. Everything is complete in my life. You know, when your life situation is entirely good and happy, you can get used to anything. I am lucky to have that. Of course, from time to time there are disagreements at home, like with my husband, for example: that he took me, or that he's this way or that way, reproaches that are sometimes still there. But when children appeared, especially our son, all of these arguments or thinking about marital love disappears, it must end. You are already physically and mentally preparing yourself for the fact that you should put all your efforts into this family, my family, to stay and that's it. For ten years my parents and sisters have been fighting me to leave Koian, to enter normal society, as I used to live, to live like they do in the city, in society. My parents come to Koian in the summer and all they see is this wildness, this stove. They see me alone sweeping, cleaning, heating the stove. They don't work that much because they have everything ready, electricity, gas, a vacuum cleaner. I understand their point of view, but my life is good, we manage sami po sebe.

Although her abduction dramatically changed her life and giving up her previous urban existence was difficult, Aigul says she has come to see life in Koian as a good alternative to living in the city:

> My husband sometimes works in the mine, and we have animals, but not enough money to live in the city. And if we take out a mortgage on a two-bedroom apartment, we will have to work to pay it down, and if we don't work, they'll take the house. For you it may seem we make pennies not money. But for us it's money! Everything is good here, we have enough of everything.

The complexity of her world view reflects the approach in Koian of making a virtue out of a vice. It's worth quoting Aigul at length to capture the multiple perspectives she has regarding her life circumstances:

> I moved in with my husband's family to Koian and became a *kelin* [daughter-in-law]. I had to do everything around the house – clean, cook, serve tea, and be quiet and respectful. It was a very difficult transition for me because I was used to the city. When I got married, for the first five years there was no

electricity in the village. Without light, it was a hellish life, but we got used to it. We would get up constantly at six o'clock in the morning, and my mother-in-law and I milked thirty cows, fifteen cows each by hand. We skimmed milk, get cream, make butter from this cream. Whipping butter is also not easy, manually. Then you bake bread, also by hand. You heat the oven by hand, then you cook dinner on this stove, then for an afternoon snack you need to heat the stove again, put the kettle on to boil. It's so much work. And besides that, there are the animals we need to help bring back to the barn.

Things changed when we got electricity because we didn't have to churn butter by hand and could boil water in an electric kettle. It's still a rural regime we follow, and there's a lot of work to be done. Life for women is very difficult, because we still cook and clean and take care of the animals. Of course, it is more difficult for men in winter than [for us] looking after the household. They have to take animals out to pasture every day. Winters are particularly harsh. And our farm is not small. It's hard to look after the cattle. And for women, of course, there are conditions on how they must act.

But you get used to everything. Today, my life is perfectly okay and I'm happy. My husband and his family have been good to me and helped me finish my education. When I had children, I focused on raising them. We also had a lot of help. My in-laws took in a child long ago and raised him. In exchange, he helps with the animals and his wife with all sorts of work around the house, including milking cows. I don't even have to tell her what needs to be done. If we ever move to the city because our children will need to go to a normal school, we'll always have him and his wife to look after the animals. It's one way to get extra money and protect our farm.

Today, we have everything. Why would I need anything else? Now that I'm older, people also respect me. Older women, especially those with children, get a lot of respect in Kazakhstan. The whole household revolves around me, and I don't have to do as much work anymore. I take care of my mother-in-law, but that just means I make tea and prepare food from time to time. Sure, it's easier to live in the city and my parents and my sister are categorically against me living in the "wilderness" of Koian. In the city there are gas stoves and vacuum cleaners, civilization. But we are fine here. We have a car and always go to the city when we want to. We never missed a single wedding or a birthday party, and every summer we take a drive to a lake.

The re-traditionalization of gender roles that favours patriarchal power dynamics is reflected in Aigul's "traditional" role as that of a *kelin*.[50] As a young daughter-in-law, she occupied the lowest position in the household, understood in contemporary Kazakhstan as a position equal to "an obedient and selfless slave that is also a family member."[51]

She assumed all housekeeping tasks (cleaning, cooking, serving family members, and showing respect to her husband, in-laws, and guests) and understood that her duty was to uphold the household's honour and never question her husband or his family. But once she gave birth to her first child, her status in the family was elevated and she had more say in the decision-making process.[52]

Although all women in Koian focus on the household, they are keenly aware that without them, the village could not exist and "the men would starve." A gendered division of labour provides the structure for life in the village but also varying degrees of esteem and status that are more fluid than they might seem. Over a period of twelve years of her marriage, Aigul gained respect and is now the head of the household, subordinate only to her husband. Because she lived in a city, received an education, worked as a teacher in Koian, and most importantly, gave birth to two children, she's seen as more cosmopolitan than other women in Koian.

Within this structure of familial roles around which homes are organized, there are things women are expected not to do. For example, they should not drink alcohol in front of elders (except during holidays and in small amounts) and never get drunk. While they do drink occasionally, it is only with other women of their same age group (and unlike with the men, I have never seen them drink in excess). Although attitudes are changing in Kazakhstan, in Koian there is also an unspoken rule that women don't smoke. When women in the village smoke (and many do), they do it as discreetly as possible when no one can see them. Cigarettes are still seen as something to be enjoyed only by men. And yet, these restrictions didn't bother Aigul or the other women I talked to. When I asked Aigul why she hides her shot glasses under the table whenever someone walks into the room, she said:

> You ask strange questions, Magda. I never even thought such thoughts – to ask myself why I do the things I do. But it's funny that to you it looks like we are hiding, like little kids. That's not the case. We are not hiding or are scared. It's all about respect, the rules of respect. We respect ourselves as women. We respect our elders, who have more respect – they drink in front of us, because we are younger and don't have as much respect. So, we don't smoke or drink in front of them. It's embarrassing for your old mother or father to see you drink. Only Russian women act like that. Many of them don't have any class.

When I lived in Koian, I also took part in the day-to-day household chores, helping with cooking and cleaning. But I was also considered to be a strange woman. For example, I drove a car. Many women in Kazakhstan don't, especially in rural areas. Although people were grateful for my shuttling services, men initially commented on my driving skills (or lack thereof in their eyes). Eventually, everyone got used to me having a car and relied on my vehicle. If a person outside the village commented on me being a "woman driver," everyone in the car who was from Koian always came to my defence. But I was strange in other ways. For one, I didn't have children despite being in my early thirties. By that time, most women in Koian had two and maybe a third. Second, I openly smoked. People talked about my smoking in hushed tones. I quickly learned that if I wanted to continue, I needed to hide it like the other women, which I did (at least for a while). In some way, Koianers helped me to quit because they shamed me for it relentlessly. In his typically parental way (that at times I did appreciate), Tursynbek made sure to tell me that I was acting "like a man" and made sure that I knew that it was embarrassing.

But since the village school closed down, Aigul observes that options for elevating one's status in Koian are shrinking, leading to thoughts of returning to the city:

> Initially I still worked at the school here in Koian, [but] then the school was shut down. My family has been fighting me to move out of Koian and live in normal society. It's too wild here for city people. My husband sometimes works in the mines, and we have enough animals to get a mortgage for an apartment. But the city is too wild for him. It's not wild for me. Maybe we'll move eventually, but someone needs to watch over the herds.

Most women in the village have had to renounce their desire for career development. Aigul continued to work as a teacher in Koian until the school shut down, and only two other women managed to keep meagre salaried jobs, even if they were far from ideal. Tursynbek's daughter-in-law, for example, mopped floors in the school for a pittance (10,000 Tenge or USD 68 per month) and her mother-in-law, Altynai, oversees the only telephone line in the village. But despite whatever attractions the city holds, Aigul appears rooted in the village, with her first concern being who will take care of their herds – as if the move to the city is only temporary and they will return.

Thoughts of the "city" function as a complex symbolic concept in Koian. In some sense, there is a generational and gendered divide to how the villagers imagine it. All older residents have no desire to be in urban areas whatsoever, as in their eyes the city is a place where crime is likely. Younger men feel differently, especially those who grew up in

Koian: they may not want to move to Karaganda, but they do enjoy going there for short bouts. For them the city is a place to visit and *guliat'* (hangout or party) for a few days here and there, but when it comes to long-term life plans, they often say they are "scared and will go hungry" if they move.

Narratives such as Aigul's offer a counterpoint perspective in terms of gender but also life experience. She had lived in urban areas before. For her, the city was cosmopolitan, something that her life in the village was utterly missing. Being in the city provided more than the opportunity to dine out or shop – it was a place to gather at someone's home with extended family networks. Women who grew up in rural areas often expressed no desire to live in urban centres, claiming that their husbands would end up as "alcoholics" (or worse, die from drug overdoses). But those like Aigul kept the ethos of the city alive in their imaginations, even as they came to terms with life in the village that gave them "everything" they needed.

The division of labour certainly keeps the village going, but there are other aspects of the gender divide that matter as well. The size of the herds determines how many people live in Koian at any given time, but how many animals you start with depends on the processes of inheritance. The animals and property pass to the youngest son following a system of ultimogeniture. As the youngest, he is the one who always remains in the village. Older sons can choose to stay but must establish their own herds and their own households, which is exceedingly rare because there is no surplus of housing. As there would be nothing for them to do as an occupation without displacing someone else, rather than becoming a burden in the form of just another mouth to feed, many choose to move to the city instead. Yet as shown above, their prospects in the city are not much better than at home, and their lives are still subsidized by the efforts of the villagers.

Conclusion

There is no doubt that the implementation of economic reforms following the breakup of the Soviet Union created a multiplicity of new articulations of the modes of production and ways of being in the world. Indeed, the creation of an entirely new economic system fostered new power arrangements in which the emergence of well-connected *nachal'niki* (bosses) took managerial positions in industrial enterprises, and former Soviet elites emerged in leading business roles.[53] Koian exists at the intersections of what their thoughts, actions, and circumstances show to be three paths: agricultural development, nuclear

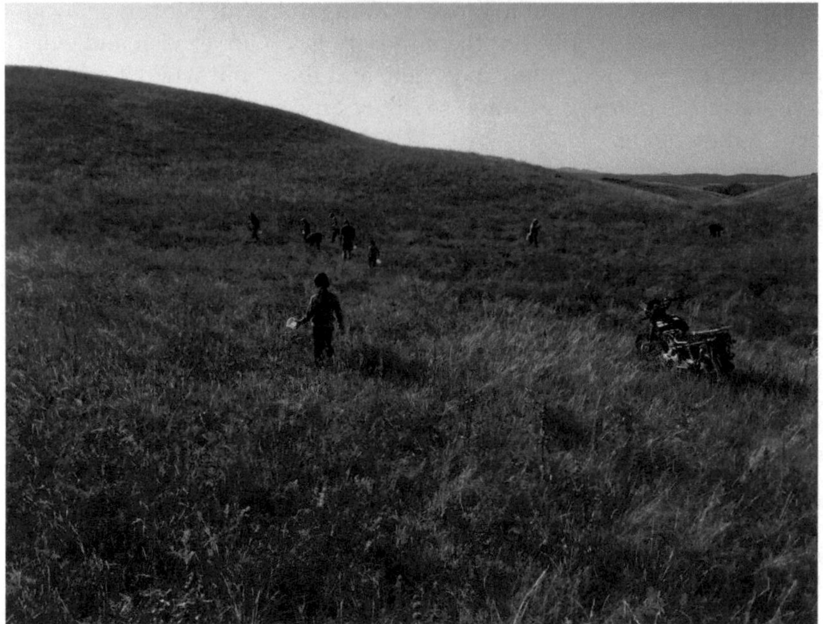

Figure 3.5. *Wild Strawberry Season*. Koianers picking wild strawberries in shallow valleys. These strawberries grow throughout this region, are used to make jams, and are sometimes used as a sugar substitute for tea.

testing, and the near-complete withdrawal of the state. The villagers who remain in Koian continue with stockbreeding while their children go to Oktiabr' or Karaganda and live with relatives to be able to go to school. Animals raised on the test site stock urban bazars, making the "disaster landscape" intimately tied to the workings of nearby cities. They are sold to provide for living expenses in the city, while the village remains central to a broader understanding of family life. It is to the village that people go to visit aging parents and grandparents – where families gather and share in what people believe is a "better life."

Capturing the challenging situation Koianers and their families in the city find themselves in, Tursynbek remarked:

Times were better during the Soviet Union. But what does one compare this to? After the fall it was worse. It's getting better now, as they say. Now everyone just wants to buy our animals and metal for cheap and make a profit by selling it for a much higher price. They take our diesel and never

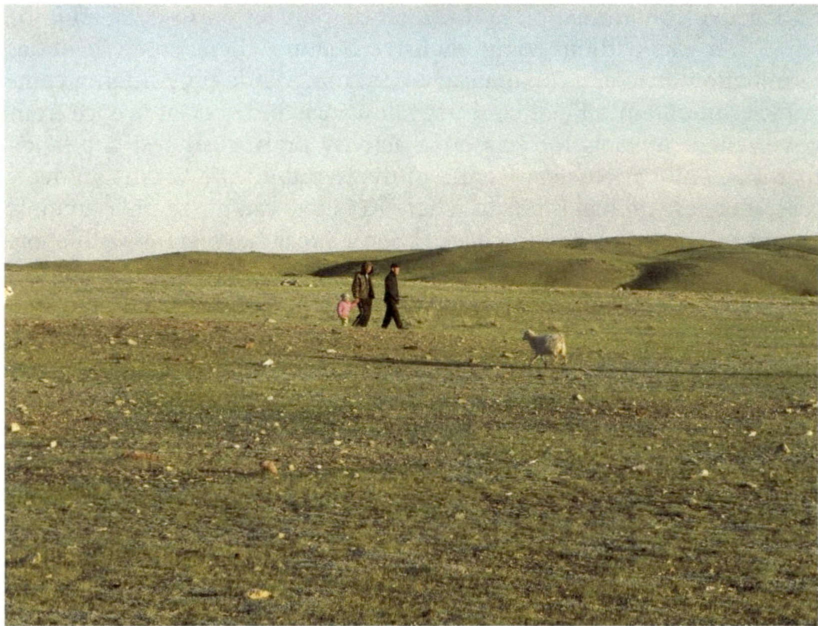

Figure 3.6. *An Evening Stroll*. After a long day's work, Koianers often unwind by walking around, catching up on village gossip and conversation.

bring it back or pay us. They make us work for nothing at these awful mines, using old machinery like in the days of gulag labour camps. On top of that, if we are not happy about work in the mines, they tell us to just quit – that they have no problem firing us and finding someone else who would be very happy to have a job.

But we don't really care. We are self-sufficient and don't live in poverty. We live sami po sebe and live simply and quietly. We are self-sufficient because our food supply grazes on pastures. It's our bank. Outsiders don't care about us, but at least the [government] administrators allow us to have this land in and around the Polygon, so we have access to good land for pasture.

As Tursynbek observes, there is no prohibition on entering the Polygon, and people have in the past received official permission to graze animals there, but what goes unsaid is the fact that there is no legal term for the Polygon. While Article 143 of the Land Code prohibits any economic activity on the land plots that have been exposed to excess radioactive contamination and cannot be transferred to ownership or temporary use without comprehensive cleanup, there isn't a legal determination of where the nuclear test site is. While only mining companies can obtain official land use allowance and special licence from government officials for economic activity on nuclear test site lands that the National Nuclear Center of the Republic of Kazakhstan oversees, there are no real limits to where Koianers can graze their animals because there is no one to check.[54] Some areas have signs with short text that walking and riding in the zone were prohibited, but this is not described in any legislation. The Polygon is therefore an economic grey zone where Koianers can pursue their collective economic activities without interference.[55]

Koianers have made a virtue out of their post-Soviet joblessness by embracing the free market opening of the Polygon as a profitable territory, despite clear risks in that proposition. And unlike in urban settings in Kazakhstan and in the communities around Chornobyl (Chernobyl) or in the US where citizens demand help for resettlement and other interventions from the state, Koianers make no such claims.[56] So far there has been not a single appeal to the court from citizens living in potentially dangerous places for resettlement. All people want is to be left alone. The choice not to demand state intervention – economic development, medical care, radiation monitoring, and so on – appear to be acceptable, normal, a matter of course, as if the options of protesting or petitioning simply did not exist. Sami po sebe is a particular form of claimlessness, an accommodation to the stripping away of rights to property, state services, and safety. It is not a collective portrait of a disposable people created by the neoliberal state. Instead, it's about people who are pioneers of a new kind of social contract that harkens back to seventeenth- and eighteenth-century social forms, where the state leaves people to cheerfully fend for themselves.

The realities of the village resist a simplistic synthesis of pastoral/bucolic reverie on the one hand and a hopeless resignation on the other. Although situated on the periphery, Koian is tied into various city networks, and despite the seeming lack of a system, the residents do, in fact, observe one and work it. Throughout my fieldwork, I shuttled countless numbers of sheep, goats, and cows between Koian and Karaganda. Together, we visited family, friends, and doctors in adjacent villages or in the cities. In all, people refused to give up living in Koian and made sure that the village was tied to Oktiabr' and Karaganda through established social networks, as well as by placing demands on the Oktiabr' akim. But people's refusal to give up on the village meant that their lives were often cut short. Some individuals died from diseases like cancer or other so-called "natural causes." Others died from suicide or from freezing to death or falling off a roof. Some even believe there was a murder.[57]

Yet even while life in Koian is fraught with difficulties – perhaps unimaginable to those who live in their urban cement blocks – for village residents this rural life, even with its limited access to food and electricity, is a better alternative. After all, would their life really improve living elsewhere? Those living in Koian insist there is a history and logic to their abandonment by the Kazakh government. Making sense of the post-Soviet reality, many people choose to live sami po sebe.

4 "They Think We Are Stupid": Reinventing Kazakh Tradition

It is so much simpler to bury reality than it is to dispose of dreams.
– Don DeLillo, *Americana*

Introduction

As a token of gratitude for help with my fieldwork, in June 2011 I took several Koianers on a vacation. I had heard about a spa several hours from the village and had enthusiastically embraced the idea of going. Set in the mountains, this pleasant *sanatoriia* (health resort) was initially constructed during the Soviet era as a holiday and medical treatment destination for families employed in the coal mines of the Karaganda region. Privatized in the post–Soviet era, it now caters to mostly middle-class Kazakh and ethnic Russian city dwellers, including miners, who visit year-round. All guests are treated to breakfast, lunch, and dinner every day. Amenities include an indoor swimming pool, sauna, table tennis, billiards, tennis and volleyball courts – even a dance hall. There are hiking trails woven throughout the grounds, a ski complex nearby, and a well-maintained beach at the edge of a small lake for swimming and small boat rentals. It was by far the most luxurious accommodations I would encounter in my decade's worth of visits to Kazakhstan and among the most revealing experiences as well.

Luckily, the decision about who should join me was not difficult to make. Children were not permitted as guests, and the village elders – several of whom had travelled quite extensively when the Soviet Union existed and the state had funded vacations to Moscow or even Prague – were simply not interested in leaving the village. This left just Aigul and her husband, Rasul (Tursynbek's youngest son) and his wife, as well as Yermek (Ramazan's son) and his wife – none of whom had ever visited an all-inclusive resort before.

The seven of us were excited to go. Gearing up for the trip, the women doubled up on their work, gathering extra water and frying extra bread to last the household for a couple of days. They coloured each other's hair in shades of red and brown and discussed which cocktail dresses, jeans, sweaters, stylish flats, and other outfits to take with them. The men did extra shifts taking out the animals. They made sure to shave and packed their nicest slacks and jeans for the trip. All of us piled into the Delica and cruised down the steppe road singing Russian and Kazakh pop songs all the way to our destination.

A People Apart

Visiting the resort solidified an inkling that had already begun to form in my mind: people from the Polygon region not only stand out (even among the same ethnic group and class of people) but are actively shunned by outsiders (including other Kazakhs). Aside from the people being considered uneducated, uncouth, and "backward," the region carries its own significance. Those coming from the Polygon frequently bear an additional geographic stigma of being polluted, biologically degenerate, and ill. Some of the reasons for this are thanks to messaging that came from the state level back in the early 1990s with regard to the legacies of nuclear testing, which, in effect, opened the door to a variety of sympathies but also various forms of social discrimination.

Ready for a weekend out of the village and dressed in knock-off Prada, Gucci, and Dolce & Gabbana, the Koianers were sniffed out by the resort staff straight away. Immediately upon our arrival, the entire staff acted as if "alerted" to our presence – not that we didn't give them reason to pause. When our group stepped towards the front desk, the staff paid close attention, fearing what must have looked like from their perspective a motley bunch that would later brawl. The men in our group were whooping and jostling each other for fun, despite the protestations from the women in the group to be quiet. After this display, the staff's reaction was predictable – when the men demanded that their small bags be taken up to their rooms and they be treated with respect like everyone else – the staff simply scoffed at them. Instead, the two front desk employees accompanied by a security guard told us to *uspokoit'sia* (calm down) because there are "other guests trying to enjoy the quiet" and threatened to throw us out of the resort if we didn't comply.

The staff watched us like hawks throughout our stay, treating us like we were juvenile delinquents and repeatedly instructing us to behave ourselves and enjoy a *short* stay. Under their watchful eyes, the Koianers' demeanor was perceived as being "off" in other ways besides the males' roughhousing. The villagers were often told to lower the volume of their speech, to walk and not to run through the courtyard, and not to monopolize the whole dance floor with their moves. Their cosmopolitan countrymen also whispered behind their backs about the cheap jeans and sunglasses they wore together with brightly coloured polyester shirts. Guests at a neighbouring table at the banquet hall (where assigned seating is standard) openly mocked the difficulty some Koianers had eating with forks (which they typically don't use at home). Members of our group were repeatedly approached, asked where they were from, and told bluntly by hotel staff and patrons alike that "we know who you are, and we don't want any *svoloch'* [scum, riffraff] here."

Class distinctions have sharpened in Kazakhstan since the Soviet collapse, with the Koianers perceived by both the staff and the urban clientele as "rural bumkins"[1] that were too "backward" to be allowed to participate in "civilized" holiday activities the resort offered.[2] Although the resort is far closer to Koian than cosmopolitan Karaganda, it is not typical to find rural people there, and especially not from the Polygon region. It was an expensive experience, one geared for middle-class urban dwellers and to whom the staff accordingly caters. In the eyes of the clientele and staff, the villagers had neither the social, cultural, nor economic capital to gain their acceptance.[3] The post-Soviet class gap characterizes a "social apartheid" of sorts, where rural populations are excluded from experiences the middle- and upper-classes enjoy.[4] The paler patrons of Russian descent seemed all too willing and able to meet and socialize with one another as guests on vacation. Urban Kazakhs – identifiable by their highly proficient Russian – were also accepted. But the Koianers were a people apart. Responding to both subtle and not-so-subtle signs of unwelcomeness, they were happy to stay to themselves.

Like the clientele at the resort, urbanites mostly speak Russian (considered an upper-class language before the Russian invasion of Ukraine in 2022), are usually economically well off, and are highly mobile. They hold a barely restrained contempt for rural populations when the latter attempt to mix with city folk and generally believe in the words of anthropologist Saulesh Yessenova[5] that "villagers should stay in the village where they belong, have skills suitable to dealing with the rural environment and production, and will be happier there than in the city anyway." How the Koianers were perceived and treated carries over from culturally introduced notions of modernity stemming from Soviet-era colonial rhetoric about "archaic" and "primitive" rural life.[6] When Kazakhstan saw a large influx of people into cities during the post-Soviet period, a geographic divide hardened into a rigid social distinction that continues to impact popular thinking about ethnicity, culture, and status.[7] Since then, urban elites have reclaimed and redefined what rural is. Unlike the villagers from Koian, they are at liberty to move back and forth, into and out of what they perceive to be "nature," as they like.[8] But the villagers from Koian, seen as trapped in their rural lives, were treated at the resort as the ultimate "other" – childish, unprofessional, and "alcoholic" village dwellers.[9] Had their patched-together and dust-covered Lada and Neva cars been strong enough to make the trip, they would have been easily spotted in a parking lot otherwise full of imported Toyotas, Audis, and Mercedes.

The treatment of Koian residents at the resort offers a vivid example of how rural Kazakhs represent an unacceptable level of cultural difference – one that is out of place in a "cosmopolitan" setting. Such social encounters can and do underscore obvious levels of abuse and discrimination. At the resort, the staff and city guests performed their own culturally informed perceptions about the village folk. But from the moment we checked in, I wondered why Koianers were not equally upset about their treatment. For example, I discovered that the momentary embarrassment some of the women felt when checking in wasn't directed at the behaviour of their partners but "offered" on my behalf. Conversations after the fact revealed no other moments of self-consciousness occurring to them that might have checked their behaviour in search of acceptance. Not only did the Koianers manage to have a tremendous amount of fun during our three days at the resort, but no one complained about being shunned. Everyone seemed to double down on acting in a way that signalled "backwardness." Koian men repeatedly ignored staff warnings to be on "good behaviour" and instead partied loudly outside, jumped rambunctiously into the pool, and danced the nights away. They spoke Kazakh as loud as they could, making fun of other patrons, knowing that much of the staff and resort guests, many of whom were Kazakh themselves, were probably unable to speak it fluently (if at all). As I came to understand, their jubilant attitudes, paired with the linguistic clash created by their native tongue in an otherwise Russian-speaking venue, was something they were proud of.

Upon our return, I spoke with Tursynbek about our experience at the sanatoriia. He enjoyed recollecting our stay and offered the following reflection:

> Everyone who doesn't live in Koian, including the people from Oktiabr' who themselves once lived in Koian and are our relatives, think we are stupid. Most people don't know where we are on a map. People from Oktiabr' know that Koian is their ancestral home but still think of us as living in *zhopa mira* [the ass of the world] when they move out.

But not content to leave matters there, he went on to explain who the *truly* backward people were:

> Kazakhstan is the only country that brings in *tupoi* [ignorant] people. The *oralmany* who came from Mongolia and settled in Koian for a while were so backward that the first time they saw noodles, they ate them dry. They drank tea with salt and lived in yurts. The family slept together and went to the bathroom together. They lived in the zimovka on the Polygon and got rich by growing a large herd. They moved away because Koian is not their ancestral home. But we stay because it's our duty. It's where our ancestors are buried, and we are mostly free to do what we want.

Tursynbek's take on the cultural differences between the Mongolian oralmany revealed an important aspect about their village identity – everyone it seems has a "backward" person they measure themselves against. Even the rural Kazakhs from the Polygon – viewed by segments of the wider society to be "genetic mutants" and "social outcasts" – situated themselves as superior to someone else as a way of maintaining esteem in the difficult post-Soviet landscape.

Ironically, and despite evidence to suggest otherwise, people who live in the cities generally perceive the Polygon populations – with their access to free land, their alleged ability to invest all of their capital in the supposedly gigantic herds, and their access to metal – as rich. When I frequented Karaganda during fieldwork, people often spoke to me of the villagers living near the nuclear test site as *Poligonskie* (of the Polygon) and as *bogatye* (rich) and therefore not in need of special treatment or government assistance.[10] Perhaps judging from the cramped and deteriorating apartments in Karaganda typified by Soviet-style khrushchëvki,[11] villagers on the Kazakh steppe could be taken as wealthy (although this perception contrasts sharply with the everyday reality of living in the nuclear zone and rural areas more generally). Although the Polygon is indeed an economic asset, the money made in the former sovkhoz is simply not enough to allow most people to move to the city or significantly improve their standard of living. Yet the mental picture of rural wealth that some city dwellers have, coupled with a general contempt for rural communities, adds to their further marginalization.

There are countless examples of social discrimination, stigma, and marginalization that people from Koian experience at regional hospitals, schools, public institutions, and elsewhere. NGO workers have done little to assuage this, describing Polygon residents as generally "uneducated and stupid" (albeit "rich"). In Karaganda, I observed some of the younger villagers being treated as thieves, as well as berated and pushed around by urban residents. Anthropologists and philosophers have long observed that social labels and stereotypes can shape an individual's identity and behaviour, leading to a self-fulfilling prophecy.[12] But what is remarkable is how Koianers respond to such characterizations. There is an admitted boldness and pride in their manner when speaking of such experiences outside the village – an attitude that captures the way in which their perceived marginalization has helped them to see themselves (unlike their urban countrymen) as the *wisest* of Kazakhs.

For example, consider the meaning of "backward," which has several connotations of interest here. On the one hand, it can obviously denote a lack. On the other hand, it means a direction. Koianers often cite the importance of their cultural ancestry as a reason not to move from the area, preferring to stay in what they call "Koianistan," a place they consider ancestral, with its own land and rules, more desirable than any other village, town, or city elsewhere in Kazakhstan.

Given how Koianers are treated by outsiders, there is no question that confining themselves to the village is the most liberating thing they can do and something almost natural. "The people who are older here, our age [mid-30s], they won't go anywhere because it's their way," Aigul remarked. "They were born here, and their descendants lived here. But even though younger people can and often leave [us] elders, we will stay and live out our lives here. It's hard to live elsewhere." Although Koianers consider what they do a "return" to the lives that their ancestors led, they have, in fact, altered the Kazakh migratory tradition of moving across an annual route paying respects to ancestors buried in many places, re-creating ancestral duty as staying put.[13] The village is both where these veritable "outcasts" can live where their roots are without experiencing the multitude of stresses that encounters with the outside world provide.

What I came to learn is that Koianers' *refusal* to feel stigmatized, demeaned, and even excluded by others at the resort – their individual and collective actions to reject the legitimacy of the authorities and outsiders – allowed them to simultaneously reject and embrace post-Soviet hierarchical social relationships.[14] As anthropologist Carole McGranahan put it, "To refuse can be generative and strategic, a deliberate move towards one thing, belief, practice, or community and away from another."[15] In other words, to refuse is to say "enough"[16] – "we refuse to continue *on this way*."[17] Whereas resistance describes opposition to direct domination, refusal is a disavowal of power relations.[18] Refusal is the Koianers' *affirmation* of their lives as they have chosen to live them.

How has refusal become part of Koianers' relational strategy? What kinds of negotiations must they make with the outside world and with themselves? Where do they draw the line, and why? What are the consequences of insisting that village life and their way of doing things is better? I want to focus next on two particular kinds of social interactions – with the scientific community and the medical establishment – that have hardened the Koianers' refusal of the way things are done outside the village and led them to affirm their own system.

Experimental Rabbits

Koian may be distant and isolated, but it is not hidden. For some in the global scientific community, Koian is an interesting place from which particular kinds of knowledge can and have been obtained. In 1997 the International Association for the Promotion of Cooperation with Scientists from the Independent States of the Former Soviet Union (INTAS) funded a research project on the Polygon.[19] The primary purpose of the INTAS research was to carry out an extensive study on the relationship between radiation exposure and the high incidence of cancer found among people living in a region.[20] What was initially supposed to be a two-year assignment turned into a three-year endeavour that included a multinational team of thirty scientists – toxicologists, epidemiologists, biologists, radio chemists, and other experts from Belgium, France, and Kazakhstan. Weighing their options among the numerous settlements near the Polygon and working in consultation with Semyon's ecological centre, the team decided to study Koian, selecting another settlement more than one hundred miles (160 kilometres) east of Karaganda as a control area.

From a scientific point of view, the setting was compelling. The people in Koian were a veritable "virgin population," never studied before in such a way. Its geographic proximity to high concentrations of lingering radioactive pollution – plutonium, strontium, caesium, and americium – with generations of people born and raised in one location made the village a perfect research site. Indeed, some of the scientists began to think of Koian as a natural laboratory of sorts, populated by ideal research subjects – "willing" and "docile" in their words – ones they assumed would be easy to work with. Beginning in the summer of 1997 and for three summers thereafter, this rural corner of the country became a centre of what seemed to many of its residents at the time a fervent scientific activity and investigation.

In short order, one hundred women and ninety-five men (including forty-seven children below fifteen years of age), all ethnic Kazakhs living in Koian, were enrolled as a study population to answer larger questions about the effects of radiation exposure on human and animal biology, as well as the environment. For the researchers to learn about potential intergenerational differences, the population was divided into three subgroups: (1) people born before 1949 (i.e., before the beginning of nuclear testing), (2) those born between 1949 and 1963 (i.e., during the period of atmospheric nuclear testing), and (3) those individuals born after the 1963 Limited Test Ban Treaty prohibiting testing in the atmosphere and underwater (i.e., individuals not directly exposed to the dispersion of radioactivity from atmospheric tests). For four consecutive summers, various biospecimens – blood, stool, urine, and sperm – were collected and shipped to a university in Karaganda for analysis. The study also examined the biological circulation of radioisotopes by taking food, animal bones, manure, and other samples, as well as by examining birds (house sparrow, rock dove, and the common wheateater), mammals (red-cheek ground squirrel), fish (wild carp), and reptiles (sand lizard). Soil, sediment, surface and groundwater, and wild plants were also evaluated. Over the course of the study, it became clear (at least to the scientists) that Koian's residents were ingesting significant amounts of radioactive elements such as plutonium, strontium, and caesium. Their genetic parameters also showed statistical differences between exposed and control groups concerning chromosomal aberrations (dicentrics, single fragments) and increased genomic instability (comet assay). The final report offers the following stark revelation:

> The most remarkable effect is the very high increase (by a factor of 7, $p < 0.001$) of the observed frequency of dicentric chromosomes (considered a reliable indicator of radiation damages) in the [Koian] population.

In addition to more frequent chromosomal aberrations than any other group, small children and men especially showed higher concentrations of radioisotopes in their bodies. Unlike women (who spend most days at home), children and men inhale soil particles because they spend more time outside. It remains an open question in the final report whether these visible molecular effects were a result of present chronic radiation exposure, inherited from higher exposure at the time of the weapons tests, or were the cause of illnesses such as cancer.

Despite the inconclusive nature of the findings, the INTAS study was dubbed a success. One epidemiologist reminiscing about her time in the field said the following to me one afternoon in 2012 over tea: "We all became good colleagues – the scientists that is. We went to conferences together, published papers, and I was able to finish my dissertation using data I collected in Koian." When I met up with her again in 2019, she noted enthusiastically that her work and career were going well – in no small part because "we collected so much information that most of us are still using it to write articles." But none of the copious amounts of data or the final study results were ever shared with people in Koian. In fact, no one in the village learned from the scientists that people there suffer higher rates of cancer than elsewhere in Kazakhstan or that they are literally eating radionuclides.

From a scientific point of view, Koian residents were abstracted into desirable human subjects and didn't "need" to be informed about the details of the study. This was a widely shared sentiment, perhaps best voiced by Boris, an epidemiologist working on the project who I interviewed in 2012:

> Koian was perfect. Three generations of people lived there while the Soviet Union tested its nuclear weapons. Since the fall of the Soviet Union, no one ever came to this village, so people welcomed us with open arms. They were happy, calm, and easy to work with. The residents thought we were medical doctors, but we told them that we were there to just study them. But they didn't really understand that we were advancing scientific knowledge on radiation and not there to provide medical care. There was a medical doctor [Nurzhan] working in Koian and she helped us convince the villagers to participate in the study. Whatever she ordered them to do, they did without question. She had lots of authority. Because of her, we were able to collect feces, sperm, and blood, but didn't give people information. This is because if you tell them the truth about what we eventually found they wouldn't understand anyway – they are not educated. We gave her the results and we don't know what she did with them. Maybe the villagers would try to petition the government for compensation, but our data would not be good enough to prove that they are sick. Plus, what can we tell them really? We did the analysis. We found plutonium where a lot of horses graze. One hundred percent there is cesium, plutonium, and other elements. We saw that people have internal exposure to radionuclides. And there's accumulation of these elements in people's bodies. But people live there, have animals, everything is open, and no one does anything about it. We don't have any power to do anything. We protected them because there is no cure for what ails them. We can't give them drugs or tell them to stop eating their food or stop living on polluted land. They are happy as is – why should we scare them?

This paternalistic approach towards individuals living in Koian allowed the scientists to focus their energies elsewhere – namely, collecting various biospecimens necessary to complete their study. The bodies of seemingly marginal Koianers became evidentiary devices that could be scientifically and socially seen[21] – but not by Koianers themselves. Susanne Bauer,[22] a science, technology, and society scholar with a background in environmental epidemiology, explains that in post-independence Kazakhstan, "the mutations detected at increased frequencies among exposed populations in the vicinity of Soviet nuclear facilities" commonly led to the "mobiliz[ation of] international resources, concern and specific funding slots for radiobiological and epidemiological studies." However, none of the mobilized resources were ever used to help Koianers improve their health and well-being. The scientists working in Koian paid only a small fee to Nurzhan, who became a local interlocutor and who helped them get the research study properly off the ground.

Nurzhan's participation was key to the project's success, and in 2015 she explained her role to me as follows:

> When I worked for INTAS, I was bringing them people. My job was to get everyone to agree to participate in the project. I also helped the villagers answer questions – the scientists needed me to help them with the questionnaire surveys that all study participants had to complete. This was probably the most important part of the project because data from the questionnaires allowed scientists to evaluate the health status of the population. I knew Koianers' medical histories, so I could help. I frequently had to remind the villagers that they were sick from this or that, because they didn't remember or didn't want to say or were too embarrassed.

A local physician and a respected member of the community, Nurzhan had two main responsibilities in the INTAS study. First, she was tasked with convincing Koianers to join it, which didn't prove very difficult because the villagers had a deep respect for her. Koianers often spoke of her as a competent doctor who was able to properly treat their injuries or illnesses. With her help, all forty-eight families (totalling 195 people) who lived in Koian at the time of the study agreed to participate.

Nurzhan's second job was a bit more difficult, but one that made her indispensable to the study. She was to make sure that Koianers responded truthfully to questionnaire surveys about their living habits and health conditions. Nurzhan knew a lot about life in Koian and had access to everyone's medical histories. Everyone in Koian completed the surveys in her presence during personal interviews. But her role in the study as a mediator between the villagers and the scientists was complicated:

> All the documents I got from INTAS were lost somewhere. I didn't share anything with [Koianers] because it's not like they would understand the results of the study. Even if Koianers would get the information about the study findings, people will never move out of Koian. You'll have to kidnap their parents when they're still alive. If they die there [in the village], no one will move. Some people have two cows, that's it, but they sit there barely scraping by because their ancestors are buried there. I'm glad that my sister and brother live there for good. They must take care of their health. They won't move to Oktiabr' because there are problems with [access to] water and they would have no access to fruits. In Koian there are strawberries everywhere in the summer and we can always visit with family. It's nice to visit the village, our ancestral lands.

Despite being a Koianer herself, Nurzhan saw no need to share the findings with them, claiming they would "never move" anyway. But her attitude reflects the larger and more complicated history of Koian – one that included villagers' positionality vis-à-vis the "outside" world and how they navigate their own health, cultural ways, and economic strategies. She understood them to be people who would simply accept their lot as both victims and agents of their own social, political, and economic displacement. If people caused problems for the scientists, she feared, local officials may punish the villagers by not plowing the road or with threats of resettlement. Her explanation for how things are in Koian seemed to give her permission not to share the study findings as if she was protecting them.

From the mid-1990s onward, Cold War and Western scientific practices took on a hybrid form. With the help of the European scientific community, Koian residents were reimagined on a molecular level and subjected to what sociologist Nikolas Rose[23] calls the "politics of life itself." They became the targets of novel forms of authority, expertise, and bioeconomic exploitation.[24] In the first decade after the end of the Cold War in Kazakhstan, the extraction of human biospecimens allowed for the examination of radiobiological processes at the cellular scale.[25] At the same time, however, the specimens gained use-value by entering the free market, where they were circulated between various national and international laboratories, analysed, and used for publication. Yet even while their specimens travelled – the products of coercive methods of research conduct and data collection – Koian residents' names were kept confidential in seeming accordance with Western scientific protocols protecting study populations. Paradoxically, as the scientific and economic use-value made the biospecimens visible, it rendered the people of Koian "invisible or unrecognizable"[26] as victims of Soviet-era nuclear testing.

The INTAS study and its approach towards Koian residents was not new. In fact, the international team of scientists from the INTAS group closely mirrored their Soviet predecessors in not bothering with "informed consent," meant to protect any human subjects in research but especially vital in work with vulnerable populations. Soviet scientists also began a project working there in the mid-1950s, with many of the same assumptions and expectations, practices, and behaviours. The Polygon was considered sparsely populated by the so-called "uncivilized" natives, and thus its residents were perfect research subjects, ordered out of their homes during nuclear tests, while information collected about them was kept secret. Soviet-era scientists also collected various biospecimens from the residents while they conducted their own top-secret human radiation studies directly ordered by Moscow. The architects of the Soviet nuclear bomb project wanted to know what sort of damage their weapons caused to the human body. From 1956 until perhaps as late as 1989, Soviet physicians travelled from one Polygon village to the next, collecting blood, feces, urine, and other samples, in addition to recording illnesses found.[27] During these comprehensive health surveys (the 1958 expedition was the largest in scope), the radiological situation was studied in almost all settlements where radiation fallout was recorded. In one regard, however, the Soviet scientists did differ from the INTAS scientists; while neither offered real medical care to the residents, at least the Soviet scientists offered vodka.

Although history shows that the Polygon and the many who live there are not new subjects of research, the collapse of the Soviet system and the near collapse of science in Kazakhstan underscores one other difference in the Polygon's evolution as a research site. The biologists that remained in Kurchatov and Semey were forced into the market model and had to look for their funding. If their research produced tangible results in the form of dissertations, peer-reviewed articles, and more research questions, their work would beget other funding. Unlike the Soviet scientists who were generously funded by the state, entrepreneurialism is a necessity for scientists making their careers anew out of a former research site that they actively help to maintain.

False Compliance

Koianers were fully aware of being perceived by the INTAS scientists as living in a village that no one visits in a frontier wilderness. They also knew they were culturally coded, both by local and international experts working there, as "backward," "uneducated," and otherwise unassuming. The INTAS work was still vividly remembered in Koian when I arrived years later to start my fieldwork. Ramazan often spoke about the study but as an elder often put it in context: "We've been experimental rabbits for half a century. We can't say no or who knows what will happen. We must *ne shumit* [not rock the boat or make noise]." From his perspective, if they were to cause trouble, the akim could refuse to plow the road or some high-level government official could show up and yell at them, leading to even further difficulties. Most of the residents I spoke with who unwittingly participated in the study have come to believe that the scientists misled them, forced them to give "embarrassing" fluids and products from their bodies, and failed to inform them about investigation results.

That doesn't mean, however, that everyone always acquiesced to what was asked of them. Through forms of obstruction, whether refusal, false compliance, or lies, villagers performed acts of refusal that are rooted in the historical record of Koian's geography and intersections with what are now multiple levels of scientific research. In as much as their behaviours appear to be affirmations, they have nevertheless come to internalize a dynamic that hedges the respect and fear they have for the medical and scientific establishment by refusing to comply in the small ways that they can, illustrating their agency in the face of a systemic power differential. Ramazan illustrated this attitude in remarks about the INTAS researchers:

> The doctors came to Koian all the time. The new ones that came after the test site was closed asked us for sperm, blood, and feces. Sperm! Can you imagine that? What would they want with sperm? They told us that they wanted to see if it was strong and if we will have children. We have children so who cares? Obviously, we are okay or else the doctors would say something, and then we could obtain compensation from the state. But not everyone gave them sperm. People refused. And we also didn't tell them everything. We just watched and laughed when they went to the outhouses to collect our *fekaliia* [feces].

The compensation program Ramazan refers to was established in 1992 and was designed to provide medical and financial assistance to victims of Soviet-era nuclear testing. One requirement of this program that would provide additional compensation is that victims must offer evidence of their victimhood – not just proof of a domicile near the Polygon at the time of testing but proof of illness (determined by a special council) associated with radiation exposure. Because the INTAS study was not directly shared with Koian residents (or could show causation), no one in the village was able to use the findings to advocate for themselves even if they wanted to. Yet as Ramazan points out, Koianers refused to participate in the study in a variety of ways and found amusement in the lengths to which the scientists would go to collect evidence from their experimental subjects.

Aigul, reminiscing about the INTAS study, offered additional examples of the ways in which Koianers refused to comply:

> We live next to the test site, but we don't really know anything. It does not depend on us. What can we do? We don't feel anything about [the Polygon], no one instilled fear in us, we don't feel this fear at all. We even go and collect metal there. How much metal, how much cable we collected! And I remember the study. [The scientists] came and took sperm from men. I don't know why, but they took it. Many men decided to go work the fields instead of staying in the village. Men who went to get hay didn't give them anything. But some of the men gave sperm. Do you know why they took it? I think they wanted to check the sperm – if it's alive, not alive, that's what it is, right? For the guys it's a joke, they're crazy, you know. And no one seriously says anything, why is it, how is it. Did you get the result? I am embarrassed to ask men this question. Yeah, I am ashamed, and I wasn't interested later. We all laughed, and then we left it like that. But we also lied [to the scientists] about things. Everyone lies in Koian.

INTAS questionnaires sought to collect a variety of personal and medical data. People were asked about their marital status, family structure, living conditions, work, monthly income, education status, food consumption, and lifestyle habits and history of diseases. Aigul and other women in the village I spoke with told me they didn't really want to participate in the study or to provide truthful answers to the questionnaires. They were self-conscious and ashamed about certain aspects of their personal lives. Despite Nurzhan's presence when filling out their answers, the research findings from the questionnaires reflect their refusal to tell the whole truth. For example, all women interviewed said they did not smoke (and never have) – despite many of them smoking occasionally and some on a regular basis. Most also claimed they never consumed alcohol, whereas in fact the women drank regularly (albeit never to excess like the men).

Men, on the other hand, were self-conscious about their personal medical history and tried to avoid revealing it. Tursynbek offered this characterization of the surveys:

> We didn't tell them anything and they [the researchers] didn't have many of our records. Men don't go to the doctor. Nurzhan was the one to tell them things like if we had the flu or experienced headaches, even when

we forgot we had this or that disease. She also exaggerated how sick we are. It's probably because she thought we would get compensation for being sick from testing. But we didn't want her to say anything because we know we're not going to get compensated. We could even lose our jobs.

Tursynbek's answer reveals that rather than seeking the status of a victim, he and others were particularly keen to be portrayed as healthy.[28] Kazakhstan's Labour Code requires medical examinations as a condition of employment in certain occupations.[29] For employees working in food, healthcare, or educational fields, as well as occupations in which physical ability is essential to the work to be performed (like mining or other dangerous work), annual medical examinations are required as a condition of employment. Tursynbek and others wanted to avoid any negative consequences that could have arisen from divulging information that could prove to be detrimental to their employment in the long run. Part of their fear comes from not knowing whether the results would become public – indeed, not knowing in general what would happen with the data at all.

Suspicions of the medical establishment run deep in Koian, and the reasons people don't seek treatment or then lie to doctors when they do cannot be separated from systemic abuses that many of them have experienced. The INTAS study is part of the larger picture. It's an all-too-common refrain that villagers are not treated seriously as a matter of geography. The Polygon has doomed many of them to shortened lives of ill health. In important ways, they have internalized this and sought their own cures and explanations for sickness and disease, and many of their conditions go undetected as a result. But the healthcare system that they've come to know has always been unreliable, leaving many to see it as a poor choice. Choosing to participate, the villagers believe, is to take one's life into one's own hands. Many simply refuse.

A System in Shambles

Perhaps the most vivid story I heard about the villagers' attitude towards the medical and scientific establishment involved another kidnapping. Tursynbek recounted the event to me as follows:

When Rasul [Tursynbek's son] was ten years old, he fell hard on his back playing outside. It later swelled up into this huge lump. We eventually had to take him to a nearby hospital to get help because he couldn't walk straight and was hunched over all the time. We were worried. But the doctors immediately diagnosed him with *kostnaia tuberkuleza* [bone tuberculosis] and wanted to do some sort of back surgery. I thought it was a *sumasshedshii diagnoz* [crazy diagnosis]. You don't get tuberculosis by falling. And spine surgery is dangerous! It could leave Rasul paralyzed because these doctors don't know what they are doing. They are not trained. Many people go to hospitals to get help but end up dead instead. To them we are all just Poligonskie, so there is no cure.

In Koian, it is a widely held belief that hospitals are not to be trusted. Reports of misdiagnosis and unnecessary treatments have fuelled the local rhetoric that "hospitals are places to get killed." As a result, alternative healers who practise outside the biomedical approach to health are favoured over traditional medical facilities:

So, in the middle of the night, me and one of my friends decided to break into the hospital and spring Rasul out. We kidnapped him! It was so brave of us to do that! We were like warriors. From the hospital we went straight to a *znakhar'* [healer] and she cured him! He was fine in two weeks. The healer is also an *iasnovidets* [clairvoyant] and can help women during pregnancy, properly diagnose people, and can tell who stole horses or find missing people.

During my time in Koian, I had the opportunity to visit one such healer in the company of Altynai, her daughter, and the daughter's in-laws. The healer's husband told me that she discovered her talents in 1986 when she began hearing the voices of ancestors during her walks through the cemetery. To maintain her focus and energy, she adheres to a strict regimen, avoiding anything that might dirty her, such as cleaning a fireplace. Her reputation as a successful clairvoyant has earned her the respect and high status of not only those seeking treatment but also government officials.[30] Tursynbek shared that she was even consulted in the case of a kidnapped government official's son, who was ultimately found.

If Koianers were simply ignoring the benefits of modern medicine, their refusal would be easy to dismiss as a form of "superstition." But in many respects, any benefits from the medical establishment have not reached the rural interior of Kazakhstan. During the Soviet era, Kazakhstan's healthcare system was state run. It was called the Semashko model of socialist medicine, one centrally planned and hierarchically organized.[31] The Semashko system was intended to provide universal access to healthcare for all citizens and emphasized preventive care (especially with regard to communicable diseases) and public health. As a multi-tier system, care was organized around a network of hospitals, polyclinics, and other secondary and tertiary units.[32]

During the Soviet era, Kazakhstan experienced persistent shortages of medical supplies, equipment, and trained personnel. Rural areas suffered from limited numbers of healthcare workers and polyclinics offering basic medical services such as vaccinations, diagnostic testing, and treatment for common illnesses. The focus on preventive medicine and public health meant that patients with serious illnesses or chronic conditions like diabetes or cancer did not receive the same level of care as their urban counterparts. Although the original drive was to develop a rural primary healthcare infrastructure throughout the Soviet Union, by 1970 the focus had shifted to specialist work and hospitalizations and away from primary care. Resources for healthcare declined overall in Kazakhstan in the 1980s, only to implode in the 1990s with the dismantling of the public health sector.[33]

Since the collapse of the Soviet Union, Kazakhstan's healthcare system has been subjected to various reforms. It faced significant challenges, including financing, medical expertise, and medical supplies.[34] Today the system operates as a mix of decentralized public and private institutions with government financing and regulation. The Ministry of Health oversees the provision of medical services and regulates the country's hierarchically organized healthcare sector, with oblast' health departments managing all state-owned clinics and hospitals and delivering healthcare services in their jurisdictions.[35] Under this system, most citizens have access to basic medical services through government-funded programs that can be supplemented with available private insurance. Out-of-pocket payments for patients account for nearly 40 per cent of total healthcare expenditures in Kazakhstan, much of it for drugs.[36]

In recent years, the government has made efforts to modernize and improve the healthcare delivery systems, especially in rural areas. Despite reforms, entrenched challenges remain in delivering effective medical care in remote regions.[37] It's a particularly notable continuity with what came before during the Soviet era; and as before, an emerging "double burden" of chronic and infectious diseases, co-epidemics of tuberculosis, HIV, and AIDS, but also chronic cardiovascular diseases, diabetes, and cancer pose significant threats.[38] To exacerbate these problems, between 2013 and 2018, over 50 per cent of rural hospitals were closed.[39] And although Kazakhstan has 407 physicians per hundred thousand population (significantly higher than the WHO European Region average), there is an acute shortage of doctors in rural areas, as well as adequately trained nurses and other medical specialists.[40] Perhaps unsurprisingly, the lack of healthcare workers is most pronounced in the northern regions of the country in places like Koian.

Today, Koianers lack access to healthcare facilities of any sort, since a nurse who lived in the village has recently left. According to Koianers, she lacked an adequate supply of drugs and "proper training" because "she bought her diploma." Most Koianers did not trust her and rarely sought her help. The only drugs she had available were *novokain* (novocaine) and *kal'tsiia* (calcium) supplements, both of which were expired and useless for treating even a small infection. Interestingly, these same drugs were sometimes used to treat ailments that don't respond to these drugs, like stomach cramps, for example.

The nearest hospital is situated 150 miles (more than two hundred kilometres) away. As is often the case in rural areas throughout the country, this hospital is in poor condition. Despite its sixty-five-bed capacity, it caters to a population of 39,455, of which 9911 are ages zero to fourteen. Medical services are limited to laboratory analysis, X-rays, ultrasounds, electrocardiograms, and endoscopies, and while it does have a maternity ward and some surgical capabilities, complex treatments such as cancer or tuberculosis can only be accessed in Karaganda. Paid medical services include *medosmotr* (medical examinations required on an annual basis for police officers and those working in food production or dangerous jobs, among others), physical therapy, and dental services. With 446 staff members, including forty-four doctors, the hospital is understaffed in terms of pediatricians, general practitioners, and obstetricians. The hospital also oversees ten outpatient clinics, nine obstetric clinics, and thirty-four rural outposts, some of which (like the one in Oktiabr') may only have a single nurse or room available to serve the community.

Similar to what he says of lawmakers in the country, Tursynbek insisted that the state of medical expertise is to be doubted at every turn.[41] Hospital and rural health clinics are staffed by people who "bought their diplomas" and "don't know what they are doing." He explained further:

> The level of medicine in this region is horrible. If we do end up in the hospital, they just tell us we are Poligonskie and there's nothing they can do. They'll kill you. The doctors can't diagnose and don't have drugs anyway. They prescribe vodka! So, we ask them – should children drink vodka too? We can make our own medicines or get antibiotics or whatever we need from Nurzhan. Women go and give birth there, but that's mostly it. It's best to avoid that place or any clinics. We can buy medosmotr. If we didn't, none of us would be able to get a job even if we wanted to.[42]

Like many other men in Koian, Tursynbek seldom visits a doctor. In fact, examining the dispensary journal from the rural clinic in Oktiabr', which records the types of care sought and the corresponding conditions, no men from Koian is listed as having sought care at the clinic between 2008 and 2011 (the years covered by the journal).

I wanted to know more about why people from Koian avoid contact with the medical establishment. In 2011, I interviewed the hospital's deputy director for medical work. Dastan was eager to chalk up the reluctance of Koianers to their "mentality":

> We service areas within a radius of two hundred kilometers [125 miles]. We have many specialists and offer good care. We can treat bronchitis, appendicitis, heart attacks, and accidents, and send serious cases to Karaganda. We even have a mobile Roentgen [X-ray] unit that drives around all the villages once a year, but the people just tell us they don't want us there. Their mentality is that way.

The "mentality" of Koianers was raised as an issue in many conversations I had, offered as a catch-all explanation for the recalcitrant ways in which Koianers behave. It's offered up as an obvious truth, as if rural people lack the critical thinking skills necessary to evaluate something as important as their health, without any consideration about the quality of care they receive or their experience in general with the medical establishment.

At a regional hospital, I asked Dastan about the possible treatment options available to people who live near the Polygon. At the same time as claiming that residents were fine, he complained that the "aul'skie [backward village people] know that medical care is free in Kazakhstan, so they don't take care of their health until it is too late." He subsequently admitted that his view drew upon what he knew of the American for-profit healthcare system in which people seemingly seek medical care all the time and thus are persistently in good health. My conversation with him concluded with a remarkable admission on his part. In all seriousness, Dastan opined, "Of course they are sick. They are from the Polygon. But they can prevent serious radiation-induced illness completely by drinking fifty or a hundred grams of vodka." Dastan was not the only doctor I spoke to who cited Soviet military studies (none of which I was able to locate) claiming vodka protects against radiation. This belief is widely held, and I was routinely advised to drink vodka when driving around the Polygon. At one of the mines I visited with Tursynbek where he worked, instead of respirators and protective clothing, the workers were given one litre of vodka that they eagerly consumed in full before beginning work inside a dusty open excavation pit. Like Dastan at the hospital, the mine operator cited

Soviet medical studies that prove vodka protects against radiation. On the Polygon, vodka seems to have replaced the need to establish a system of radiation monitoring or adequate healthcare. It has become a "bad faith" cure to a problem of toxic realities people find themselves in and a passive acceptance of the status quo.[43]

The belief in vodka's ability to protect against radiation exposure might be seen as a convenient illusion when dealing with health issues on the Polygon. To drink from a bottle when returning home is a local remedy to avoid confronting the true extent of environmental and human harm brought about by decades of nuclear testing in the region. In "Americana," Don DeLillo explores escapism as a coping mechanism in a world of individual alienation, dominated by the harsh realities of consumerism. Similarly, on the Polygon, vodka is an escapist coping mechanism, a way for people to deal with uncertainty. Embracing alcohol (and inebriation) as a solution to many health problems people face, some in the medical establishment are choosing to "bury reality,"[44] inadvertently perpetuating a cycle of denial and complacency surrounding a radioactive legacy that has become a problem that's too big to fix.

I asked Tursynbek about vodka. "Who knows. Maybe it works, maybe it doesn't work against the *radioaktivnye mikroby* [radioactive microbes]. Vodka is great for taking the edge off, for not having to think about anything. So in a sense it's a cure." The ready acceptance of vodka as a palliative might appear to confirm Dastan's assessment regarding the mentality of Koianers. But a little probing revealed a different attitude. The fact that Koianers see through the medical establishment's condescension was neatly if frighteningly captured by Tursynbek's reaction when we discussed what Dastan had said. "What about the children?" he yelled, becoming enraged as he contemplated the medical advice Dastan dispensed. "Are they supposed to become alcoholics? What about women who are pregnant?" he raged, calling Dastan a corrupt apparatchik who only cares about *den'gi v karman* (money in his pocket). Upon calming down, he admitted that at his advanced age, "I can't drink like that any more." Clearly, he retained a sharp sense of his own agency in medical matters.

Conclusion

Altynai's and Aigul's list of undiagnosed health problems includes bone pain, kidney and stomach problems, and constant headaches. Both know they suffer from chronic anaemia. But none of their symptoms have ever been properly diagnosed by a healthcare professional. Aigul explained:

> They just want us to pee in a cup and tell us we have protein in our urine.
> I think this means our kidneys are failing. And then nothing is done be-
> cause we are from the Polygon. The nurses are afraid to talk to us about
> the Polygon because they don't want to become *vrag naroda* [enemy of the
> people/state]. So, they treat us for diseases that are not there and don't tell
> us anything. A woman in Oktiabr' was diagnosed with breast cancer and
> ended up at the local hospital, where she stayed for two days without any
> help. They didn't have morphine and didn't offer care. And they didn't
> want to take her to a Karaganda hospital even though they are supposed
> to. No basic care at all.
>
> Everyone's bodies hurt in Koian: kidneys, head, stomach. All the kids
> are slower, less sociable. All women have anaemia. When our children get
> bronchitis and we happen to be in the city, we'll go to this dog restaurant ...
> dog meat is good for that. We know how to help ourselves. We have only
> physical work, no mental work like you [Magda], so our bodies hurt.

The one time I visited a hospital with Altynai, she was prescribed a combination of aloe vera and honey for her painful migraines. Justly sceptical, on the way back to Koian, we stopped to visit the healer, who prescribed a secret concoction of herbs that seemed to work wonders for Aigul's headaches.

It's not surprising that most people in Koian rarely visit a doctor and prefer to avoid them if they can. This larger healthcare picture – the lack of transparency, inadequate treatment options and incompetent doctors, the cost and scarcity of medicines, the mandatory yearly medical check-ups for those working in the mines, and the marginal status of Koianers in the eyes of the medical establishment – translates directly into a structural framework that limits access to effective medical attention.

Koian residents are part of a radiobioecological legacy that began during the Cold War and that continues to this day in which the medical establishment has never represented anything positive for them. The inhabitants of the Polygon belong to a particular landscape or "mutant ecology,"[45] coming into being with the explosion of the first atom bomb in New Mexico in 1945 and continuing across the planet and into Kazakhstan. As a result, they are also part of the practices of empire that have come to bear on plants, animals and people. As geographer Jake Kosek[46] observes, nuclear developments, whether in weaponry, energy, or medicine, "have clearly been consequential to different ecologies and species; some transformed while others are destroyed – through bombings, depleted uranium, land mines, or massive infrastructural development." The kinds of research practices undertaken by the INTAS group, as mentioned in the ecological context by Kosek, should prompt us to discuss the specific social environments that have emerged. These conversations help us get a sense of how people navigate through destabilized political, economic, and cultural landscapes.

To be "rural" in Kazakhstan is at once to be noticed when one leaves the village. Most villagers spend very little time in cities or "urban" areas, or places where "urban" people go. A system of social and cultural capital has taken shape through sets of behaviours, knowledge structures, and places (such as resorts or clubs) in which they have very little experience. In some actual sense, they are visitors from the periphery when they do appear. But there's something else too. Koianers represent a different world of sorts, a past of antiquated beliefs and economies. The ways in which the so-called aul'skie are interpreted is never positive. It has no bucolic meaning that brings to mind a hard-working ranching life. Quite the opposite occurs, where the primary association is a degenerative lack. This external perception can also be found in the ways medical practitioners and other researchers have engaged with the villagers, whether for genealogical information or biospecimens.

Koianers feel their sense of difference in their bodies and sometimes fear the violent motives that they cannot separate from Soviet-era biomedical work. But rather than show resignation, they instead refuse in the ways in which they can, even if it's just playing games with interviewers or by holding their heads high and speaking Kazakh around a dinner table full of Russian speakers. By intentionally embracing their inward-focused (but not insular) identity, claiming to prefer life in the village to elsewhere, Koianers avoid engagement with a medical establishment that sees them as less than human. By distancing themselves from mainstream society and refusing to be confined by scientific and biomedical categories in a world of limited economic opportunities, they make their own rules.

Conclusion: The Atomic Present

For anyone who has never lived in the steppe, it is hard to
understand how it is possible to exist surrounded
by this wilderness on all sides. But those who have lived here
since time out of mind know how rich and variable the
steppe is. How multicoloured the sky above. How fluid the
air all around. How varied the plants. How innumerable
the animals in it and above it. A dust storm can spring
up out of nowhere. A yellow whirlwind can suddenly
start twirling round the air in the distance in the same
way women spin camel wool into twine. The entire,
imponderable weight of that immense, heavy sky can
suddenly whistle across the becalmed, submissive land ...

– Hamid Ismailov, *The Dead Lake*

Following the closure of the Polygon in 1991, the victims of Soviet nuclear tests became (for better and for worse) symbolic capital in Kazakhstan's nation-building agenda. The human tragedy wrought by that period is indisputable. Scientists have found that the Polygon region has the highest rates of digestive cancer, lung cancer, female breast cancer, cervical cancer, and cardiovascular disease (just to name a few) of anywhere else in Kazakhstan. In that biomedical conversation, those who received particular attention from the state and the media were people living with congenital anomalies and those whose deaths were attributed to above-ground testing and the fallout from it. They became the physical manifestation of Soviet-era nuclear devastation of a region where nearly a quarter of the world's nuclear testing occurred. Local and international journalists and filmmakers covering this Soviet legacy over time have continued to add to the dramatic effect of testing from these years, frequently showcasing the anatomical museum in the Academy of Medical Sciences in Semey. There, in various mason jars, is a macabre collection of embalmed fetuses from area maternity hospitals arranged in neat rows. In one you can see a "cyclopic" foetus; in another, a two-headed creature with a tail, seemingly half-human and half-animal. The eerie display is meant to serve as a stark reminder to the world of the horrors of a nuclear apocalypse, often featured in documentaries about the Polygon. But in truth, these exhibits are more likely from all across Kazakhstan and likely date from before 1949 when nuclear testing began.[1]

The media has helped a great deal to bring the tragedy of the Polygon to the public, but it has sometimes done so at the expense of fact. The notable documentary *After the Apocalypse* (2011) by the British filmmaker Antony Butts is a case in point. Described by *The Guardian* as "a sombre, painful and sometimes almost horrifying work," the film explores the lives of a mother and daughter living in a village near the Polygon, both of whom were born with severe facial deformities.[2] The daughter, who is pregnant, faces condemnation from a local doctor who believes it should be illegal for individuals with genetic mutations to reproduce, citing studies that show the intergenerational inheritance of genetic damage caused by exposure to radioactive contamination.[3] Not surprisingly, the doctor views deformed human beings as the "face of the future" of Kazakhstan and proof of "genetic genocide" unless preventive measures are taken.[4] While this may be an understandable position in light of the Soviet government's disregard for human life, the main characters' congenital anomalies in the film are not due to nuclear fallout, as the mother was born before testing began. Nonetheless, the film's director creates the impression that the condition is directly related for dramatic effect.

I screened Butts's documentary with several residents from the Polygon region, some of whom served in an advisory capacity during the film's production. They found the whole thing quite upsetting, but not for the same reasons that I did. I took issue with the ethics of genetic passports, an overly invasive and abusive medical system seeking to control sexual reproduction, and a film director who unfairly linked the deformity of its main character to nuclear fallout. But those watching with me were upset that an elderly woman was shown visiting a nuclear crater while her son was drinking vodka to stave off radiation. I learned while screening the film that people's dissatisfaction with this representation of the Polygon victims was rooted in the fact that a community not entirely dissimilar to theirs was shown in a derogatory way and painted as a picture of a "failing" (biologically and otherwise) and "backward" society – a perception at odds with how the village residents view themselves. Their reliant attitude was summed up in a remark by a fifty-year-old resident at the conclusion of the screening: "They should make a film about how people have to plow their own roads in winter instead."

As an anthropologist, my charge is to take stories and media such as these into account when writing about the afterlives of nuclear testing in Kazakhstan. What kinds of things are being said about the people who live there? What is not said? The American writer and philosopher Susan Sontag[5] observed that images have the power to shape our perceptions of reality and are often used to manipulate public opinion. Images of the disfigured individuals from the Polygon region are frequently used for political purposes to create a sense of Kazakhstan's national unity around a communal trauma. They both reveal and conceal the reality of the suffering that residents experience and yet seemingly have had a numbing effect rather than inspiring a call to action.[6] In Kazakhstan, such images have contributed to the perception that residents from the Polygon region suffer from pathological conditions connected exclusively to past exposure to radiation, ignoring the social, political, and economic factors that place people's lives at risk in the present. This is a form of political nihilism that has compelled Koianers to refashion their lives anew in the face of catastrophe. "Everything that's wrong with us is blamed on the Polygon: anaemia, cancer, the flu, suicide, mental problems. Polygon this, Polygon that," Tursynbek said. But his rejoinder revealed how Koianers react to this narrative. "It's done. There is no more Polygon," he declared, highlighting a sense of resignation and acceptance.

Tursynbek is partially correct. During my fieldwork, I encountered a pair of Peace Corps volunteers who resided in the regional hub. Surprisingly, they were oblivious to the fact that they lived near the Polygon. When informed, they expressed dissatisfaction with their placement to the Peace Corps headquarters, but their concerns were dismissed as unfounded. The administrators refused to acknowledge any problems and accused me of being a fearmonger. They claimed that the Polygon was no longer a hazard, and even if the volunteers consumed items from the area, it posed no harm. However, the organization eventually capitulated to some of the volunteers' demands to be moved out of the path of Cold War radiation, and because of "a number of operational considerations," the Peace Corps no longer sends volunteers anywhere in Kazakhstan.[7]

My goal in this book has been to push beyond the limitations of meta-narratives about nuclear "victimhood" and environmental crisis.

Moreover, I have sought to highlight the wider significance of living in a radioactive wasteland (that doesn't look like one) and to reflect on the way that Koianers have adapted to their lives in the face of extreme hardship and tragedy. This is what they would have me tell. Despite appearing to outsiders to be stuck in a hopeless situation, they have managed to turn their struggles into sources of strength and the adversity they have endured into virtues.

And yet even I have been tempted to tell their story as one of unvarnished victimhood as seen through an "objective" perspective. Unmentioned up to this point is the vast array of crimes and suicides recorded during my time living among the Koianers. While conducting my fieldwork, I attended several funerals, where I heard stories about unexplained deaths and the rumours surrounding them. During one of my interactions, I had a conversation with a police detective who specialized in investigating various criminal cases in the region, including homicides, felonies, and a range of other offences. He mentioned that he was working on a case that involved the suicide of a seven-year-old student, which had shaken the regional town. "We have a lot of suicides here, including very old people, but it's the first time I've encountered someone so young taking their life. People drink themselves to death, and there are also cases of homicide," he said. As he handed me a copy of a crime report for the year 2010, I realized that the villages in the region experienced a significant number of tragic deaths. The report included two dozen suicides by hanging but also told of frostbitten corpses and poisoning by means of ethylene glycol (antifreeze). One particularly tragic report detailed how a man found his brother impaled on an iron fence next to the grave of their sister who died fifteen years earlier.

On the face of it, such a litany of desperation seemingly contradicts this book's central thesis of resilience in the face of adversity. There is no sugarcoating the suicides as a deeper story of refusal. But viewing such events through Western eyes as simply a chronicle of pain and victimization doesn't do justice to how the villagers see their experience – even experiences that might paint them in a "negative" light. Koianers had to be understood on their own terms, as subsequent events during my time living in the village would illustrate.

I came to Kazakhstan originally to study the children and grandchildren of Stalin-era deportations that swept up members of my family from Poland and sent them to hard labour or death, or both, in the steppes of Kazakhstan. After changing my research to the Polygon, I stumbled upon an unexpected (albeit distant) personal connection to the region. Through sheer coincidence, I met Ivan and his mother Wanda – my grandmother's first cousin – who reside in the Russian city of Rubtsovsk just across the border from Semey. Both Ivan and Wanda had worked in closed and secret cities that hosted uranium mines linked to the production of nuclear bombs detonated on the Semipalatinsk Test Site. Wanda even remembered once seeing a mushroom cloud. They regaled me with stories about the gruelling labour they endured but were quick to point out that it allowed them to survive in a harsh Soviet environment. Through them, I learned about my great-great-grandmother, who was a prisoner in a women's labour camp in Karaganda and was buried nearby in an unknown grave. Despite my initial efforts to locate her resting place, all I could find was her name etched on a stone monument to victims of gulag labour camps alongside the hundreds of other women who lost their lives.

I began my research in Koian with the goal of documenting how marginalized and impoverished communities cope with the lasting consequences of the Soviet Cold War nuclear era. However, as I delved deeper into life on the Polygon, I realized that just like the stories Ivan and Wanda told, framing my research solely through the lens of nuclear victimhood failed to capture the full picture of how people persevere – even in a remote village fraught with risks and uncertainties. Despite state abandonment and the hardships faced by Koianers, they have managed to liberate themselves from stigmatizing social, political, and economic practices that exclude them. Some outsiders, including scientists, continue to downplay the extent of radioactivity on the Polygon. Instead, they raise questions about Koianers' (and others like them) mental well-being. In this context, the resourcefulness demonstrated by the villagers is remarkable and has played a crucial role in shaping their ability to overcome challenges. Even in the face of gradually losing the basic necessities of life, Koianers do not make any demands for their rights or services as citizens. They cope with extreme adversity on their own, a reflection of a new social contract reminiscent of seventeenth- and eighteenth-century social forms in which individuals must fend for themselves. Anthropologist Anton Blok[8] observed that "radical innovators" often emerge from extreme adversity, and the people of Koian certainly exemplify this phenomenon.

Like many other marginalized communities around the world, Koianers possess their own unique "talent for life"[9] that revolves around a strong sense of collective identity and mutual support. Migration from rural to urban areas in post-Soviet Central Asia has been influenced by economic and social inequities, resulting in migrants congregating around larger cities in search of better wages and educational opportunities.[10] While remittances from urban migrants to their rural families have been crucial for their survival, the case of Koian shows that remittance flows can go in the opposite direction. Urban kin rely on the support of village family members who share resources such as livestock or use the proceeds from selling livestock to help with purchasing apartments. During the COVID-19 pandemic, the village even served as a refuge for family members fleeing the cities to avoid strict quarantine.

In the face of government neglect, absence of social safety nets, and social alienation, Koianers had little choice but to establish their own atomic collective – a makeshift camp where life, despite its myriad obstacles, seems to be worth the trouble of being lived. They are acutely aware of the challenges and hardships they face within their polluted environment, living in a permanent state of exception. Despite this and with little alternative, they recognize their fraternal way of life as preferable to the outside world, even if living in the village is more uncomfortable.[11] Outsiders often resent and envy them, believing the villagers to be wealthy yet also "backward" and living in wretched poverty. In many ways, Koian only presents advantages to the people eking out a living there, and villagers prefer to keep things as they are. Let me give one example.

In the melee of myths and realities that surround the Polygon, my words as an international researcher from an American university were shown to have weight from the start – that is, once an investigative media outlet learned of my presence in a village living without "proper" *usloviia* (conditions). As a freshly minted fieldworker eager to please my interlocutors, I was pressured from several sides to speak publicly about what I was doing. On one side was Semyon and the representatives of his organization in Karaganda, who asked me to further the cause of environmental justice in central Kazakhstan. On the other side was the akim of Oktiabr', who was eager to dispatch me to the airwaves to let the public know about rural life on the Polygon and possibly bring the state resources necessary for maintaining schools, medical clinics, and funds for a real fire brigade to battle frequent blazes that burn across the steppe. I finally gave in and agreed to an interview, thinking that perhaps as an American I would have a shot at influencing people's perception of the region and its inhabitants. I was eager to help Koianers as best as I could and naively thought I could make a difference.

I arrived at the 5-Kanal television station ready to provide a counter-narrative and focus on the things that mattered: the lack of basic resources in all village communities around the Polygon and the need to securitize most radioactive areas on the Polygon. 5-Kanal is a local television station that describes its target audience in the following way:

> The viewers of the TV channel are socially active residents of Kazakhstan, with a higher level of education and income. They have successfully adapted to modern life and succeed in it, are interested in what is happening in the country and the world and have their own position. They care about context.[12]

The fifteen-minute interview was ready for that day's evening broadcast and aired again the following morning. Responding to questions about my profession, I described what it is that anthropologists do and why I was living in a village next to a nuclear test site. I talked about the fires and emphasized the lack of doctors, nurses, and teachers in the rural areas and the myriad problems people face every day – the things I've talked about in this book. I ended the interview by briefly discussing the current scientific debates about the effects of chronic radiation exposure on the human body. I cited the INTAS research about their findings on residual radioactivity exposure and chromosomal aberrations, and how the findings were inconclusive about what these aberrations mean. Mostly what I stuck to was talking about the need to put warning signs around the most dangerous areas so that people will know to avoid them.

Initially, it seemed that everyone in Koian was happy with me discussing the village, even though they had only heard about the interview from their relatives in the city. Things changed in January 2011 when *Mutanty Poligona* (Mutants of the Polygon) appeared in a major Kazakhstani newspaper. The 5-Kanal television interview from weeks earlier was scooped and appeared in numerous print news outlets in Kazakhstan and in Russia over the next several months. My work had been sensationalized, with large swaths of the articles wholly fictitious. I had not come to Kazakhstan to find and study "mutants," as the article stated, nor had I come to collect blood and do genetic analysis. The piece was illustrated with a series of alarming if generic photographs: a deformed child, a radiation warning sign, crumbling ruins of a Soviet collective farm, and a picture of a distinct mushroom cloud rising in the distance.

Needless to say, these articles took some explaining once they finally made their way to the village several months later. Tursynbek, Altynai, and others in Koian knew that my words had been "invented" and taken out of context. But what mattered most to them was the title and the photographs. "Everyone just wants to talk about mutants, victims, and nothing else," Altynai said. "The funny thing is, we are not even considered the same kind of victims as those who live in other villages, even though we are closer to ground zero than they are." No one in the village was amused with how my good intentions in giving an interview had now spun out of control. "You made too much *shum* [noise or rocking the proverbial boat], and now the administrators are going to start talking about moving us out because we are 'victims and mutants.' You never can tell what they are going to do," Tursynbek snapped. Thankfully nothing ever came of my shum, and no one was ever harassed or forced to leave – a fact that is unsurprising given the overall attitude the government and Kazakhs generally had towards the villagers. Several months later, Koian was celebrated in a local newspaper for producing the most butter – a ploy by the akim to show how well things are actually going for everyone, even if no one produced much butter at all.

When I started working on this research, what drove me was the rather jarring reality that people can and do live in a region where nuclear testing occurred. I often heard (and even experienced) that the farther one lives from the Polygon, the more terrifying life there is imagined to be. Concerned biologists, radioecologists, physicians, members of environmental organizations, and others are rightly sounding alarms about this mostly unguarded territory of post-nuclear existence. I made sure to ask the scientists in Semey, who have dedicated their lives to studying the biological aftermath of nuclear testing, what they think about the current situation on the Polygon. I met the two experts in a verdant park in the heart of the city. As we sipped our steaming cups of tea and ordered shish kabobs (meat skewers), I asked if they had done any research about the current radiological impact on the population and if they ever think about where their food comes from. One offered the following response:

> There isn't much we can do. We know where our meat comes from, but no one tests it for radiation. There is no radiation testing station. We also know that studying residual radioactivity is too political, so we don't. But we know what we are finding with regards to the effects of nuclear testing. The Polygon region has the highest rates of cancers. There's also a lot of mental health problems, especially among descendants of people affected

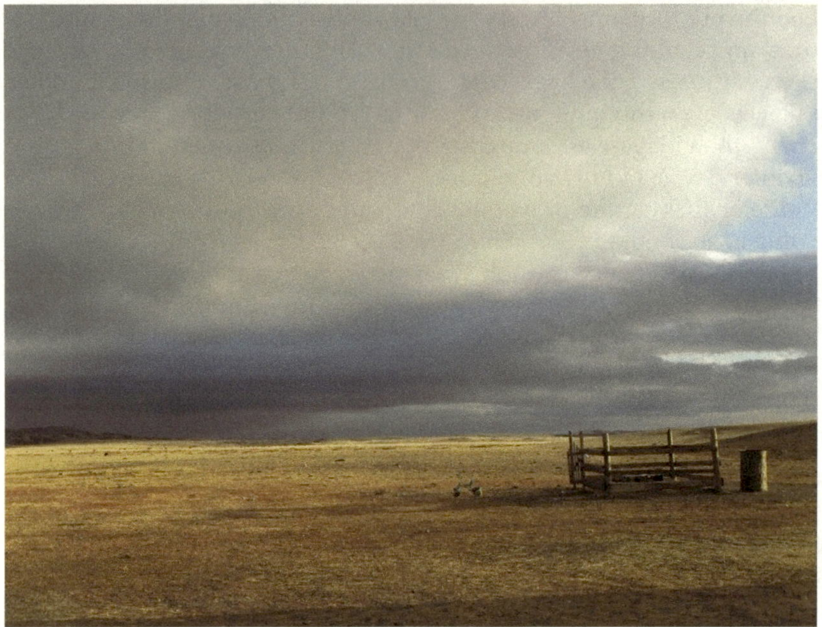

Figure C.1. *Fall in Koian*. A late fall view from my house in Koian. The ominous dark clouds looming above were a sign of the first snow to come.

by radiation, things like depression, anxiety, somatic distress, and fatigue. What is needed is social rehabilitation – psychologists who can help people deal.

Indeed, when I present my work at academic conferences or teach it in my courses, people often ask me "what should be done" about people living on the Polygon. I share their concern but recognize that framing matters in that way robs Koianers of their agency as individuals who have fashioned an existence living on the Polygon. No matter how different that life is from the life I or others lead, it cannot be denied that they are choosing the way that they can have a life they recognize as theirs and theirs alone. It's hard to imagine denying them even that much agency after everything that has been done to them.

When you ask Koianers, they are clear in their desire not to relocate because it would likely result in further impoverishment and the loss of community. They think the concerns are overblown and at a deeper level recognize that attempts to get them to move are fundamentally

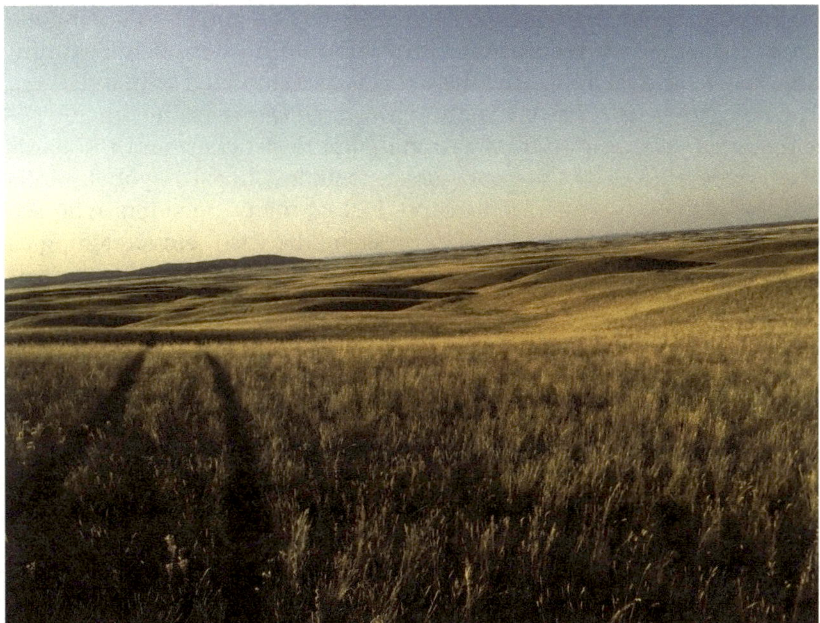

Figure C.2. *Steppe Roads*. Common steppe roads through the rolling hills of the test site.

attacks on their way of life. Standing atop a hill overlooking the village, Tursynbek declared with a sweeping gesture, "This is *nastoiash-chaia svoboda* [true freedom]." Looking across the horizon, he offered this reflection:

> It's like *dikii zapad* [the Wild West]. What are we comparing the Polygon to? The air is worse in the city. They have pollution too. Look at Karaganda, the smoke, every car releases all sorts of elements, and you inhale it. In the city, food is full of chemicals. Our food walks on the pastures. At least here we have nature and fresh air.

There is considerable truth in what Tursynbek said.

And if you asked the residents of the Polygon – the men on horseback, the cars full of people darting around on dusty tracks, and even the occasional miner trucking some kind of mineral from here to there – they would probably say the same thing. A similar attitude is captured by Hamid Ismailov in his novel titled *The Dead Lake*. The novel focuses on the consequences of nuclear testing on the Polygon by following the life of a young boy who decides to swim in a mysteriously beautiful blue lake before realizing that the water is contaminated with radiation. The boy grows up with devastating consequences to his health and social stigma. Yet despite the environmental destruction and the hardships experienced by the protagonist, Ismailov, like Tursynbek, finds beauty in the devastated landscape. Unlike many outsiders who see the steppe lands as desolate wilderness, he depicts them stretching as far as the eye can see, with its "multicoloured sky above," the "varied plants," the "innumerable ... animals in it and above it."[13] For him, like for most people in Koian I talked to, it's the stark contrasts between the devastation and the haunting beauty of the land and the life that somehow manages to thrive here that's striking.

At the same time, because locals have come to accept their situation and make no claims against the authorities, it would be very easy for the government to act like there is no need to act. The individuals of the Polygon have become accustomed to their marginal status and expect nothing as citizens of Kazakhstan. Yet to simply ignore the vast ecological and economic neglect that has been directed at the Polygon would seemingly turn a blind eye to the many deaths of despair recorded above. And yet government economic intervention in the post–Soviet era raises more questions than it offers answers to the conditions the Koianers find themselves in.

Take for example the mining industry. In the early 1990s, the leadership of Kazakhstan sought to strike a careful balance with Russia in the transfer of industrial and military enterprises and in the process secure the country's vast mineral wealth.[14] As a result, natural resource development took centre stage. By 2009, Kazakhstan became the world's primary exporter of uranium, accounting for 43 per cent of world production in 2019.[15] It also hosts the world's first International Atomic Energy Agency nuclear Low Enriched Uranium (LEU) Bank that stocks ninety metric tons of LEU hexafluoride in Oskemen (formerly the city of Ust-Kamenogorsk).[16] However, scarce state oversight and the lack of funding to deal with the inherited burden of hazardous and toxic waste from the Soviet era has been an internationally recognized problem, as has worsening environmental damage. A Human Rights Council Report[17] described Kazakhstan as "facing a situation where its natural resources and environment are seriously deteriorating across all crucial environmental standards." The nation has more than 22.3 billion tons of industrial waste (5.2 billion of which are toxic) and one hundred million tons of municipal solid waste.[18] Karaganda region has accumulated more than eight billion tons of waste, one-third of which is hazardous.

Today, millions of people live in the vicinity of abandoned or active uranium mines or countless other sites contaminated with heavy metals, radioactivity, or other invisible pollutants. Some studies suggest that forty thousand children under the age of ten years old have lead poisoning and neurological diseases as a result.[19] Of course the Polygon is just one of many problems.

Nor are other economic development plans met with enthusiasm – quite the opposite. Koianers were upset about a government proposal to lease more land around the Polygon, which would bring hundreds of horses to the area. The introduction of so many animals would have a detrimental effect on the food supply for local livestock attempting to graze on a depleted grass supply. I was even told people have resorted to setting fires to the fields themselves as a means of protest – a remarkable development no matter how you think about it.

Koian has undergone some small changes over time, but what is more striking is how despite widespread changes around the world, it has maintained the way of life I've come to know. Essential amenities such as roads, a medical clinic, a school, or even a store are still absent, and people continue to rely on livestock breeding. In 2019, the mine that offered some Koianers and others wages was closed, leaving many residents without a source of additional income. Tursynbek explained that the mine's closure was due to the company filing for bankruptcy to reduce taxes and receive a five-year tax break when they reopen under a new name. As for him, his pension has finally begun and he's happy to never set foot in a mine again. As for something additional to do in his retirement, he spoke about offering "safari" tours to the "traditional Kazakh" steppe, an idea that Semyon and others had presented on several occasions before.

Some individuals have left the village while others have arrived, including families working the land and herds of absentee city residents. I was told these workers are foreign "guest worker" types who get paid with food rations and a roof over their heads. Others struggled to follow the social expectations of the village. When I returned in 2019, I learned of a horrific suicide attempt that nearly took the life of one of my neighbours. He told me how he slashed at his throat and would have died in a pool of his own blood had the village not wrapped him up and whisked him off to Oktiabr'. He blamed his depression, loneliness, and the history of mental illness in his family. But it was the failure of his youngest brother to take over the family cattle enterprise that stripped him of the ability to leave the village like all older sons do to start a life elsewhere. He wasn't married, had no children, and had nothing to look forward to. In other words, he couldn't lead the kind of life required in Koian. In the village, people lightly shunned him for a time until he got back on his feet and kept the dream alive that he will eventually find a wife, have children, and raise so many animals that he'll be able to move to the city.

In time, I also stopped worrying about the same things that had previously occupied me – the Polygon, the poisonous radiation, or an illness that may or may not come. I had better things to do with my time – fetching water, driving to the store, cooking dinners, and stockpiling supplies – than to contemplate Soviet legacies or their consequences thereof. People continued to survive so much that the radioactivity of the Polygon seemed a small issue in comparison. I found myself even rolling my eyes at questions about victims and radiation and wanted my friends back in the United States to stop asking about my Geiger counter and instead just send me Advil and vitamins, a proper hammer, and an electric hair cutter that Koianers could really use. For everyone in the village, it was more important to have food, shelter, and warmth than to worry about the latent effects of invisible harms. And yet during fieldwork, I couldn't avoid getting drawn into conversations about the "victims" of nuclear testing and in the process inadvertently reproduce many of the narratives that already circulate about the people who live there.

My last visit to Kazakhstan during the writing of this book was in 2023 (though I returned to the site again in the summer of 2024). Several years ago, I began talking with Timothy Mousseau, a biologist at the University of South Carolina, known for his groundbreaking research involving dogs and barn swallows in the Chornobyl (Chernobyl) Exclusion Zone. Mousseau is a leading expert on the intricate workings of animal genetics. After we learned about each other's work, I invited him to come along. All was as usual in Koian. The village seemed to hold steadfast in its familiar state (with the exception that now people use motorcycles in the summer, rather than horses, to follow their animals). Not so for the Polygon, it turned out, where a whirlwind of activity was unravelling particularly in those regions that fall beyond the Karaganda oblast' boundary. The familiar winter farm outside Koian and near the atomic craters had been rebuilt. It wasn't just the new construction that was surprising on this old, abandoned spot, it was the materials. The roof was green corrugated metal, the familiar sky-blue trim of Soviet Kazakhstan was now more teal or aquamarine, and the

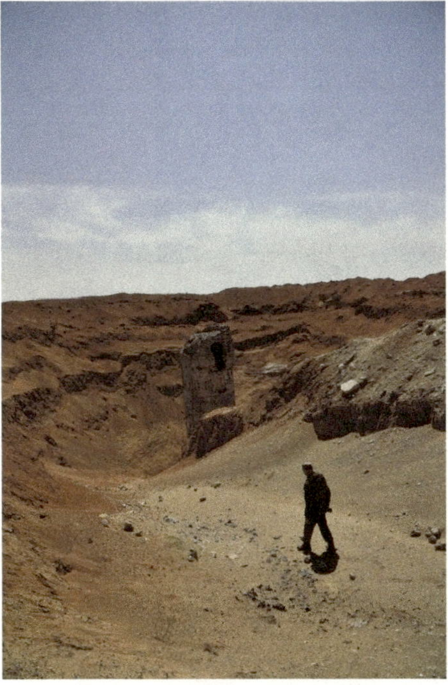

Figure C.3. *The Diggers.* Unknown diggers use machinery to excavate around what people claimed were former missile silos to extract rebar and other metal. In summer 2023, there was a frenzy of activity on the test site focused on this task.

windows were far larger. Next to the house stood a long wide barn, built for what the owner boasted were his fifteen hundred horses that gallop freely across terrain marred by craters.

Mousseau and I stopped in on every settlement on the Polygon in the summer of 2023, which confirmed a more systemic change – most of the test site was under reclamation for livestock breeding. One in particular stood out. For all intents and purposes, this was a ranch, with a brand-new house with Wi-Fi, solar, indoor plumbing, and a stockbreeder who flaunted his herd of five thousand horses. It stood adjacent to an abandoned goldmine and in proximity to areas once subjected to the testing of radiological warfare agents, which made the scene all the more unsettling. It was all utterly surprising, yet nothing prepared me for the excavations going on throughout the Polygon. Traces of tractors and

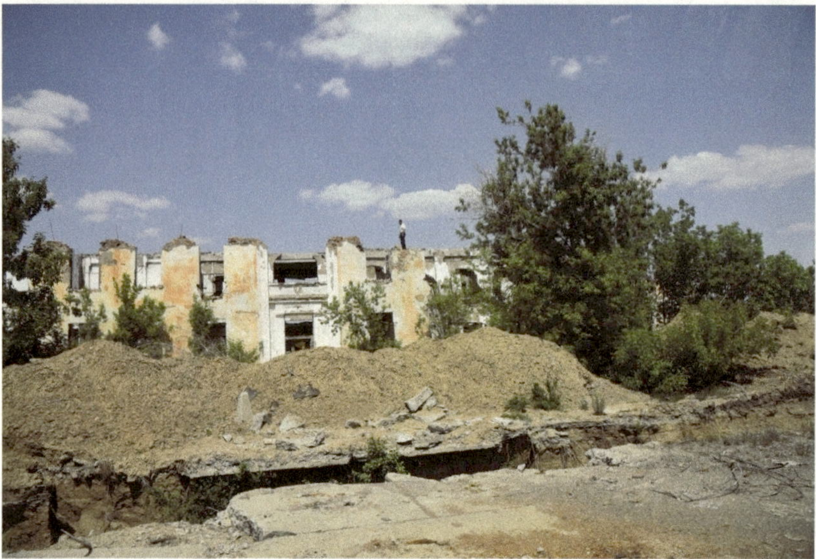

Figure C.4. *Searching for Metal*. A person on top of a hollowed-out building on the Chagan airbase that once housed planes that dropped atomic bombs on the Polygon. He is collecting metal from the walls.

dredgers were seemingly everywhere where craters or former weapons silos stood.

It all appeared orchestrated, the heavy machinery gouging and pulling at the earth, their tracks weaving in and out like a construction site. The scene looked like something out of the Arkady and Boris Strugatsky[20] novel *Roadside Picnic* where people known as stalkers illegally enter the contaminated Zone to find valuable artefacts left behind.

It was a jarring sight to see so much land disturbance occurring and quite a stark contrast to the 2023 legislation Kazakhstan adopted, supposedly aimed to create a semblance of safety around the Polygon. What we watched was like a scramble for the nuclear zone – a rush to extract every shred of metal and to stake a claim over lands deemed better suited for pasturing animals. Even the abandoned military town of Chagan saw this fervour. The landscape looked like a war zone. Entire five-storey buildings were deconstructed and toppled in piles. The runway that once served part of the Soviet nuclear fleet of aircraft was taken apart slab after concrete slab, the rebar broken free and sent on trucks driving towards Semey.

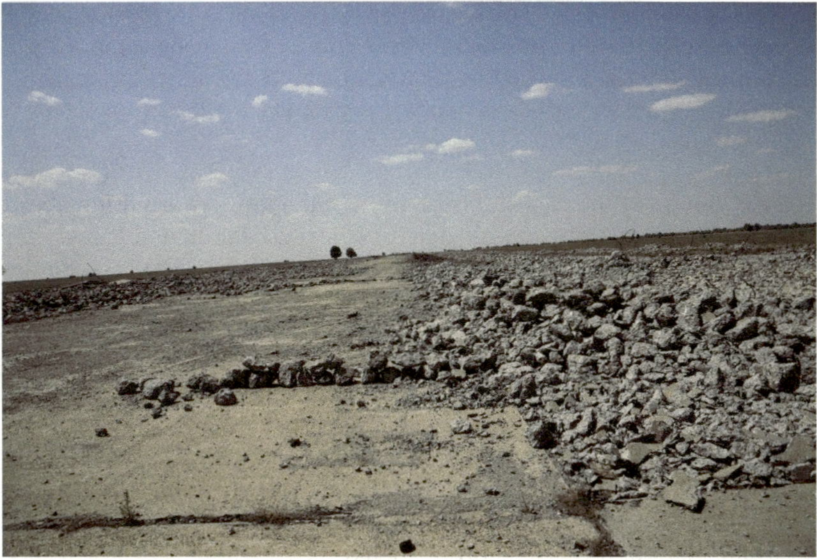

Figure C.5. *Chagan Airstrip*. Both sides of the airstrip show signs of
damage, with crushed concrete and missing rebar, likely taken by unknown
individuals and transported to Semey to be sold as scrap.

Mousseau, having spent time pouring over available scientific studies on the Polygon months prior, reflected on the situation in the following way:

> From my perspective, this atomic wasteland offers unique opportunities
> to assess landscape-scale genetic and ecological impacts of chronic expo-
> sure to a radionuclide, tritium, that has largely escaped rigorous scientific
> scrutiny. As a consequence of its unique history, this region has become
> an *unnatural* laboratory that may provide invaluable and unparalleled
> insights into the insidious and potentially eternal ramifications of ge-
> netic damage that can accrue when multiple generations are chronically
> exposed to a mutagen. Of particular concern is the possible ecosystem
> consequences of bioaccumulation and biomagnification of tritium up the
> food chain.

I spoke about the current Polygon situation with Semyon back in his
Karaganda environmental organization. Having participated in the
Parliamentary group to change what was happening, he reflected:

> This law [On the Semipalatinsk Nuclear Safety Zone] is a way to open a
> testing ground for economic activity and steal a lot of money, supposedly
> to ensure strategic security. But the worst thing for me in this law is that
> there is nothing about the safety of the population, their resettlement, or
> the cessation of grazing.

Indeed, none of the goals and objectives of the law say anything about animal pasturing or the people who live near contaminated areas.

The Polygon region has a long and complicated history of Soviet nuclear testing, and the villagers have had to adapt to this challenging environment to keep the atomic collective alive. If they commonly suffer from anything, it is sheer physical pain from the hard work that they do. It's the pursuit of making things work in this isolated village that I've tried to explain in these pages – the villagers' strategies for survival rooted in the area's histories that they know, coloured by the social, political, and economic contexts and upheavals that structure so much of their lives. Despite the difficult circumstances they face, Koianers are incredibly resourceful. They have learned to make the most of the limited means available to them, and they have developed a strong sense of community as a result. One of the most striking aspects of life in the village is the sheer amount of hard work required to keep things running smoothly. From gathering hay and collecting water to keeping track of livestock and repairing homes and fences, Koianers are constantly busy with tasks that are essential to their survival. Living in the village, I have come to appreciate the incredible strength that the villagers possess. While Koianers expose important dynamics between transnational and more local responses to questions of long-term contamination, victimhood, and how we understand and study them, in the end they are also simply a remarkable example of the resiliency of the human spirit.

Glossary of Select Terms

aul a traditional Kazakh settlement; often refers to a small village comprising extended families today

glasnost' a policy of openness and transparency

kolkhoz a collective farm

Komsomol All-Union Leninist Young Communist League

oblast' a larger administrative region containing multiple raions

otdelenie a smaller and semi-independent unit of a sovkhoz, responsible for specific land and output

raion a district of a larger administrative region

sovkhoz a state-owned farm

Notes

Foreword

1 Zhazira Dyussembekova, "Kazakh Street Artist Draws Attention to Social and Environmental Issues," *The Astana Times*, July 11, 2016, https://astanatimes.com/2016/07/kazakh-street-artist-draws-attention-to-social-and-environmental-issues/.
2 Svetlana Alexievich, *Voices from Chernobyl: The Oral History of a Nuclear Disaster* (New York: Picador, 2006)
3 Pat Ortmeyer and Arjun Makhajani, "Worse than We Knew," *The Bulletin of the Atomic Scientists*, November/December 1997, pp. 46–50.
4 Alice Callahan, "How Red Wine Lost Its Halo," *The New York Times*, February 17, 2024, https://www.nytimes.com/2024/02/17/well/eat/red-wine-heart-health.html.

Introduction

1 Jan Zalasiewicz, Mark Williams, Will Steffen, and Paul Crutzen, "The New World of the Anthropocene," *Environmental Science and Technology* 44, no. 7 (2010): 2228–31. *See* also Jacob Hamblin, *Arming Mother Nature: The Birth of Catastrophic Environmentalism* (New York: Oxford University Press, 2013).
2 Jacob Hamblin and Linda Richards, eds., *Making the Unseen Visible: Science and the Contested Histories of Radiation Exposure* (Corvallis, OR: Oregon State University, 2023).
3 Institute of Biophysics of the USSR Academy of Medical Sciences, "Vypiska iz Otchota Resul'taty Naucheneniia Vozdeistviia Radioaktivnykh Osadkov na Ob'ekty Vneshnei Sredy i Sostaiane Zdrovia Naseleniia Itogi" [The results of studying the impact of radioactive fallout on environmental objects and the health of the population]. (Archive in Semey Scientific Research Institute for Radiation Medicine and Ecology, 1958).

4 According to the Parliament of Kazakhstan data I obtained from the environmental organization in Karaganda, as of 2005, 1,323,000 people were recognized as victims of nuclear testing, and 1,057,000 received certificates confirming their "victim status." Koianers are ineligible for these IDs because they don't live in the Abai (formerly eastern Kazakhstan) region. There are no publicly available sources about the number of recognized victims. Since the main criteria for counting as a victim of nuclear testing is based on the duration and period of residence, and not everyone has registered, the actual number of "victims" is more likely significantly higher. It is estimated that some three million people have been exposed to radioactive fallout, divided between the citizens of Kazakhstan and the Russian Federation's Altai region (Saim Balmukhanov, *Medical Effects and Dosimetric Data from Nuclear Tests at the Semipalatinsk Test Site*, p. 7). The population in the path of fallout received a dose between 20 and 4000 millisieverts (see "Four Decades of Nuclear Testing: The Legacy of Semipalatinsk," *EClinicalMedicine* 13, 2019, https://www.thelancet.com/action/showPdf?pii=S2589-5370(19)30151-8). There is scant reporting on radiation exposures of military personnel, and there are no detailed accounts of accidents, deaths, or illnesses impacting military personnel. Personal accounts I collected suggest that many soldiers were exposed to radioactive fallout whether through accidents or negligence.

5 Hiroaki Katayama, Kazbek N. Apsalikov, Boris I. Gusev, Boris Galich, Madina Madieva, Gulsum Koshpessova, Asel Abdikarimova, and Masaharu Hoshi, "An Attempt to Develop a Database for Epidemiological Research in Semipalatinsk," *Journal of Radiation Research* 47, no. 1 (2006): A189–A197; Roman Vakulchuk and Kristian Gjerde, with Tatiana Belkhina and Kazbek Apsalikov, *Semipalatinsk Nuclear Testing: The Humanitarian Consequences. Report 1* (Oslo: Norwegian Institute of International Affairs, 2014). Populations adjacent to the Polygon are divided into five categories of risk, based on estimates of how much radiation they were exposed to: emergency radiation risk, zone of maximum radiation risk, zone of increased radiation risk, zone of minimal radiation risk, and territory with a reduced socio-economic status. Citizens who live in these areas are entitled to benefits and compensation. For example, some are entitled to lump-sum payment (paid only to those residing in the region from 1945 to 1965), pension top-up, or salary top-up (only for government employees), while others ar entitled to annual paid leave (only for those who continue to live near radiation risk areas and are government employees), additional maternity leave, and free treatment in sanatoria. There are no benefits for people who moved to the Polygon region after 1990.

6 Eben Harrell and David E. Hoffman, *Plutonium Mountain: Inside the 17-Year Mission to Secure a Dangerous Legacy of Soviet Nuclear Testing* (Cambridge,

MA: The Project on Managing the Atom, Belfer Center for Science and International Affairs, Harvard University, 2013); Vakulchuk et al., *Semipalatinsk Nuclear Testing*. Among them are the vertical shafts (boreholes) at the Balapan field, which are enclosed with concrete, and the designated thirty-seven-mile (sixty-kilometre) "exclusion zone" at the Degelen Mountain complex, which is fenced off and guarded by drones (Harrell and Hoffman 2013). On July 5, 2023, Kazakhstan President Kassym-Jomart Tokaev signed the law *On the Semipalatinsk Nuclear Safety Zone* (Ministry of Justice of the Republic of Kazakhstan, *On the Semipalatinsk Nuclear Safety Zone. The Law of the Republic of Kazakhstan Dated July 5, 2023, No. 16-VIII* [in Russian] [Astana, Kazakhstan: Legal Information System of Regulatory Legal Acts of the Republic of Kazakhstan, 2023], https://adilet.zan.kz/eng/docs/Z2300000016). The legislation's purpose is ensuring nuclear and radiation safety and facilitating the restoration of the territory to economic activity.

7 NNC (National Nuclear Center), Republic of Kazakhstan Institute of Radiation Safety and Ecology, *Semipalatinsk Nuclear Test Site: Present State* (Pavlodar: Press House, 2011).

8 Susanne Bauer, Boris I. Gusev, Ludmila M. Pivina, Kazbek N. Apsalikov, and Bernd Grosche, "Radiation Exposure Due to Local Fallout from Soviet Atmospheric Nuclear Weapons Testing in Kazakhstan: Solid Cancer Mortality in the Semipalatinsk Historical Cohort, 1960–1999," *Radiation Research* 164, no. 4 (2005): 409–19.

9 Normal background radiation is between 0.008 and 0.015 milliRem/hr. According to the US Nuclear Regulatory Commission (2015), an average yearly radiation dose a typical American is exposed to is about 620 milliRem per year. Half of this dose comes from natural sources such as soil, rocks (uranium), and air (radon). The other half is human-made and comes from sources such as radiation therapy and nuclear power plants.

10 Several dozen underground tests were carried out in the experimental area near Koian.

11 See Magdalena Stawkowski, "Life on an Atomic Collective. The Post-Soviet Retreat of the State in Rural Kazakhstan," *Études Rurales* 200, no. 2 (2017): 196–219.

12 Russell Bernard, *Research Methods in Anthropology. Qualitative and Quantitative Approaches*, 6th ed. (Lanham, MD: Rowman & Littlefield, 2017); James Clifford and George E. Marcus, eds., *Writing Culture: The Poetics and Politics of Ethnography* (Berkeley: University of California Press, 2010 [1986]); David Fetterman, *Ethnography: Step-by-Step* (Thousand Oaks, CA: Sage, 2010); George Marcus, "Ethnography in/of the World System: The Emergence of Multi-Sited Ethnography," *Annual Review of Anthropology* 24, (1995): 95–117.

13 Donna Goldstein, "Toxic Uncertainties of a Nuclear Era: Anthropology, History, Memoir," *American Ethnologist* 41, no. 3 (2014): 579–84.

14 To the best of my ability, I have followed the Belmont Report ethical guidelines on research with human subjects, as well as those of the American Anthropological Association. My research was approved by Institutional Review Boards of the University of Colorado Boulder and the University of South Carolina, and with informed consent from all research participants.

15 Koian means "rabbit" in Kazakh.

16 The specifics regarding the types of mines cannot be disclosed in an effort to maintain the confidentiality of local residents.

17 Adriana Petryna, *Life Exposed: Biological Citizens after Chernobyl* (Princeton, NJ: Princeton University Press, 2013).

18 Holly Barker, *Bravo for the Marshallese: Regaining Control in a Post-nuclear, Post-colonial World* (Belmont, CA: Wadsworth/Thomson, 2004); Pieter de Vries and Han Seur, *Mururoa and Us: Polynesians' Experiences During Thirty Years of Nuclear Testing in the French Pacific* (Lyon: Centre de Documentation et de Recherchere sur la Paix et les Conflics, 1997); Greg Dvorak, *Coral and Concrete: Remembering Kwajalein Atoll Between Japan, America, and the Marshall Islands* (Honolulu: University of Hawai'i Press, 2018); Barbara Rose Johnston and Holly Barker, *Consequential Damages of Nuclear War: The Rongelap Report* (Walnut Creek, CA: Left Coast Press, 2008).

19 See also Ryo Morimoto, *Nuclear Ghost: Atomic Livelihoods in Fukushima's Gray Zone* (Oakland: University of California Press, 2023). In his 2023 work *Nuclear Ghost: Atomic Livelihoods in Fukushima's Gray Zone*, anthropologist Ryo Morimoto examines the repercussions of radiation on an aging population steadfast in their resolve to stay put on contaminated land after the Fukushima nuclear disaster. This demographic stands in contrast to what Akihiro Ogawa (Akihiro Ogawa, *Antinuclear Citizens: Sustainability Policy and Grassroots Activism in Post-Fukushima Japan* [Stanford, CA: Stanford University Press, 2023]) describes as the "antinuclear citizens" – a younger and broader segment of the Japanese populace – who advocate for a nuclear-free society and envision a sustainable existence. In essence, Morimoto's focus is on the elderly, shedding light on their unique experiences amid the broader antinuclear sentiment prevalent in Japan post-Fukushima.

20 Wisława Szymborska, *Miracle Fair: Selected Poems of Wisława Szymborska*, trans. Joanna Trzeciak (New York: W.W. Norton, 2001), 44. In her poem "Children of Our Era," Szymborska suggests that politics extends beyond discourse and institutions, underscoring the interconnections between politics, subjectivity, and personal identity, down to the genetic level; see also Bruce Grant, *In the Soviet House of Culture: A Century of Perestroikas* (Princeton, NJ: Princeton University Press).

21 Paul Farmer, "An Anthropology of Structural Violence," *Current Anthropology* 45, no. 3 (2004): 305–25.

22 Robert Borofsky, "Public Anthropology. Where To? What Next?" *Anthropology News* 41, no. 5 (2000): 9–10.

23 Gabrielle Hecht, *Being Nuclear: Africans and the Global Uranium Trade* (Cambridge, MA: MIT Press, 2012); Gabrielle Hecht, "Nuclear Ontologies," *Constellations* 13, no. 3 (2006): 320–31. See also Bernadette Bensaude-Vincent, Soraya Boudia, and Kyoko Sato, eds., *Living in a Nuclear World: From Fukushima to Hiroshima* (New York: Routledge, 2022); Laura Pitkanen and Matthew Farish, "Nuclear Landscapes," *Progress in Human Geography* 42, no. 6 (2018): 862–80.

24 Christopher Robert Hill, "Britain, West Africa and 'the New Nuclear Imperialism': Decolonisation and Development during French Tests," *Contemporary British History* 33, no. 2 (2019): 274–89.

25 Ogawa, *Antinuclear Citizens*; see also Melissa Checker review of *Flammable: Environmental Suffering in an Argentine Shantytown*. https://anthrosource .onlinelibrary.wiley.com/doi/10.1111/j.1935-4940.2010.01072.x.

26 Joseph Genz, *Breaking the Shell: Voyaging from Nuclear Refugees to People of the Sea in the Marshall Islands* (Honolulu: University of Hawai'i Press, 2018); Johnston and Barker, *Consequential Damages of Nuclear War: The Rongelap Report*.

27 Javier Auyero and Debora Swistun, *Flammable: Environmental Suffering in an Argentine Shantytown* (New York: Oxford University Press, 2009).

28 Daniel Renfrew, *Life Without Lead: Contamination, Crisis, and Hope in Uruguay* (Oakland: University of California Press, 2018).

29 Petryna, *Life Exposed*; see also Robert Edgerton, *Sick Societies: Challenging the Myth of Primitive Harmony* (New York: The Free Press, 1992).

30 Following anthropologist Liviu Chelcea, I use the concept of post-socialism to explore how the past continues to influence the present, considering both spatial and temporal dimensions (Liviu Chelcea, "Goodbye, Post-Socialism? Stranger Things Beyond the Global East," *Eurasian Geography and Economics* (2023), https://doi.org/10.1080/15387216.2023.2236126.

31 Auyero and Swistun, *Flammable: Environmental Suffering in an Argentine Shantytown*; Shannon Cram, *Unmaking the Bomb: Environmental Cleanup and the Politics of Impossibility* (Oakland, CA: University of California Press, 2023); Kim Fortun, *Advocacy after Bhopal: Environmentalism, Disaster, New Global Orders* (Chicago: Chicago University Press, 2001); Kim Fortun, "Ethnography in Late Industrialism," *Cultural Anthropology* 27, no. 3 (2012): 446–64; Michelle Murphy, *Sick Building Syndrome and the Problem of Uncertainty: Environmental Politics, Technoscience, and Women Workers* (Durham, NC: Duke University Press, 2006); Linda Nash, *Inescapable Ecologies: A History of Environment, Disease, and Knowledge* (Berkeley: University of California Press, 2006); Maxime Polleri, "Post-Political Uncertainties: Governing Nuclear Controversies in Post-Fukushima Japan," *Social Science Studies* 50, no. 4 (2020): 567–88; Anna Tsing, *The Mushroom at the End of the World: On the Possibility of Life in Capitalist Ruins* (Princeton, NJ: Princeton University Press, 2015).

32 Donna Goldstein, "Invisible Harm: Science, Subjectivity and the Things We Cannot See," *Culture, Theory and Critique* 54, no. 4 (2017): 321–29.

33 Soraya Boudia and Nathalie Jas, eds., *Powerless Science? Science and Politics in a Toxic World* (New York: Berghahn, 2014); Kate Brown, *Manual for Survival: A Chernobyl Guide to the Future* (New York: W.W. Norton, 2019); Donna Goldstein and Magdalena E. Stawkowski, "James V. Neel and Yuri E. Dubrova: Cold War Debates and the Genetic Effects of Low-Dose Radiation," *Journal of the History of Biology* 48, no. 1 (2015): 67–98; Lisa Onaga, "Measuring the Particular: The Meanings of Low-Dose Radiation Experiments in Post-1954 Japan," *Positions Asia Critique* 26, no. 2 (2018): 265–304; Nicolas Sternsdorff-Cisterna, *Food Safety after Fukushima: Scientific Citizenship and the Politics of Risk* (Honolulu: University of Hawai'i Press, 2019).

34 Joanna Mishtal, *The Politics of Morality: The Church, the State, and Reproductive Rights in Postsocialist Poland* (Athens, OH: Ohio University Press, 2015); Petryna, *Life Exposed*; Michelle Rivkin-Fish, *Women's Health in Post-Soviet Russia: The Politics of Intervention* (Bloomington, IN: Indiana University Press, 2005); Robert Kopack, "Rocket Wastelands in Kazakhstan: Scientific Authoritarianism and the Baikonur Cosmodrome," *Annals of the American Association of Geographers* 109, no. 2 (2019): 556–67.

35 Susanne Bauer, "Fallout Memory Trajectories at Semipalatinsk: Reassembling the Post-Soviet Past," in *Tracing the Atom: Nuclear Legacies in Russia and Central Asia,* ed. Susanne Bauer and Tanja Penter (New York: Routledge, 2022), 196–216; Cynthia Werner and Kathleen Purvis-Roberts, "After the Cold War: International Politics, Domestic Policy and the Nuclear Legacy in Kazakhstan," *Central Asian Survey* 25, no. 4 (2006): 461–80; Cynthia Werner and Kathleen Purvis-Roberts, "Unravelling the Secrets of the Past: Contested Versions of Nuclear Testing in the Soviet Republic of Kazakhstan," in *Half-Lives and Half-Truths: Confronting the Radioactive Legacies of the Cold War*, ed. Barbara Rose Johnston (Santa Fe, NM: School for Advanced Research Press, 2007), 277–98; Cynthia Werner and Kathleen Purvis-Roberts, "Cold War Memories and Post–Cold War Realities: The Politics of Memory and Identity in the Everyday Life of Kazakhstan's Radiation Victims," in *The Anthropology of the State in Central Asia*, ed. Madeleine Reeves, Johan Rasanayagam, and Judith Beyer (Bloomington: Indiana University Press, 2014), 285–309.

36 Catherine Alexander, "A Chronotope of Expansion: Resisting Spatiotemporal Limits in a Kazakh Nuclear Town," *Ethnos* 88, no. 3 (2020): 467–90, https://www.tandfonline.com/doi/full/10.1080/00141844.2020.1796735.

37 Jeanne Féaux de la Croix, Irina Arzhantseva, Jeanine Dagyeli, Eva-Marie Dubuisson, Heinrich Härke, Beatrice Penati, Akira Ueda, and Amanda Wooden, "Roundtable Studying the Anthropocene in Central Asia: The Challenge of Sources and Scales in Human-Environment Relations,"

Central Asian Survey 41, no. 1 (2021): 180–203; Botakoz Kassymbekova and Aminat Chokobaeva, "On Writing Soviet History of Central Asia: Frameworks, Challenges, Prospects," *Central Asian Survey* 40, no. 4 (2021): 483–503.

38 Sharad Chari and Katherine Verdery, "Thinking Between the Posts: Post-colonialism, Postsocialism, and Ethnography after the Cold War," *Comparative Studies in Society and History* 51, no. 1 (2009): 6–34; see also Liviu Chelcea and Oana Druta, "Zombie Socialism and the Rise of Neoliberalism in Post-Socialist Central and Eastern Europe," *Eurasian Geography and Economics* 57, no. 4–5 (2016): 521–44; Stephen Collier, *Post-Soviet Social: Neoliberalism, Social Modernity, Biopolitics* (Princeton, NJ: Princeton University Press, 2011); Natalie Koch, *The Geopolitics of Spectacle: Space, Synecdoche, and the New Capitals of Asia* (Ithaca, NY: Cornell University Press, 2018); Mishtal, *The Politics of Morality*.

39 William Wheeler, *Environment and Post-Soviet Transformation in Kazakhstan's Aral Sea Region: Sea Changes* (London: UCL Press, 2021); see also Serguei Oushakine, *The Patriotism of Despair: Nation, War, and Loss in Russia* (Ithaca, NY: Cornell University Press, 2009); Mathijs Pelkmans, *Fragile Conviction: Changing Ideological Landscapes in Urban Kyrgyzstan* (Ithaca, NY: Cornell University Press, 2017); Madeleine Reeves, *Border Work: Spatial Lives of the State in Rural Central Asia* (Ithaca, NY: Cornell University Press, 2014); Douglas Rogers, *The Depths of Russia: Oil, Power, and Culture after Socialism* (Ithaca, NY: Cornell University Press, 2015).

40 Elana Resnick, "The Limits of Resilience: Managing Waste in the Racialized Anthropocene," *American Anthropologist* 123, no. 2 (2021): 222–36; Wheeler, *Environment and Post-Soviet Transformation in Kazakhstan's Aral Sea Region*; see also Renfrew, *Life Without Lead*.

41 Livia Monnet, ed., *Toxic Immanence: Decolonizing Nuclear Legacies and Futures* (Montreal: McGill-Queen's University Press, 2022).

42 See Kate Brown, *A Biography of No Place: From Ethnic Borderland to Soviet Heartland* (Cambridge, MA: Harvard University Press, 2004) for a discussion of weak state structures in the Kresy region (now part of western Ukraine).

43 Giorgio Agamben, *Homo Sacer: Sovereign Power and Bare Life* (Stanford, CA: Stanford University Press, 1998).

44 Genz, *Breaking the Shell*.

45 See also Sharon Stephens, "The 'Cultural Fallout' of Chernobyl Radiation in Norwegian Sami Regions: Implications for Children," in *Children and the Politics of Culture*, ed. Sharon Stephens (Princeton, NJ: Princeton University Press, 1995), 292–318.

46 David Graeber, "Culture as Creative Refusal," *Cambridge Journal of Anthropology* 31, no. 2 (2013): 1–19; Carole McGranahan, "Theorizing Refusal: An Introduction," *Cultural Anthropology* 31, no. 3 (2016): 319–25.

Chapter 1

1 Keith Basso, *Wisdom Sits in Places: Landscape and Language Among the Western Apache* (Albuquerque: University of New Mexico Press, 1996).
2 In the early sixteenth century, what is now Kazakhstan was inhabited by three nomadic *juz* (hordes), or confederation of allied clan groups – the Lesser, Middle, and Great. These alliances are believed to have emerged to safeguard the steppe territories from hostile attacks, forming loose political and military unions (Martha Olcott, *The Kazakhs* [Stanford, CT: Stanford University Press, 1995]). Led by individual khans, these hordes constituted themselves as allied clan groups, each occupying distinct geographic territories but uniting for various purposes such as defence, politics, or trade. Despite their differences, all members who made up these sociopolitical groups were one people – Kazakh in language, tradition, and law (Virginia Martin, *Law and Custom in the Steppe: The Kazakhs of the Middle Horde and Russian Colonialism in the Nineteenth Century* [Richmond, VA: Curzon Press, 2001]). The Middle Horde occupied the central and northeastern pasturelands of Kazakhstan, today the oblasts (administrative regions) of Karaganda, Abai (East Kazakhstan until June 8, 2022), Pavlodar, and Akmola. Koianers were often proud to trace their ancestry to the Middle Horde but blamed atomic testing for destroying Kazakh intellectual life. They frequently spoke of the last great Kazakh poet, philosopher, and intellectual, Abai Kunanbaev and his wife, who were born nearby. A celebrated composer of traditional Kazakh music, Tattimbet Kazangapuly, has a fifty-foot (fifteen-metre) statue commemorating his life adorning his burial site a few hills over from Koian.
3 Cynthia Werner and Holly Barcus, "The Unequal Burdens of Repatriation: A Gendered View of the Transnational Migration of Mongolia's Kazakh Population," *American Anthropologist* 117, no. 2 (2015): 257–71. There is some flexibility in Kazakh kinship relations, especially relating to marital domicile.
4 Adeeb Khalid, "Backwardness and the Quest for Civilization: Early Soviet Central Asia in Comparative Perspective," *Slavic Review* 65, no. 2 (2006): 231–51.
5 Carole Ferret, "The Ambiguities of the Kazakhs' Nomadic Heritage," *Nomadic Peoples. Special Issue: Heritage Process among Nomadic Pastoralist Groups in Muslim Contexts* 20, no. 2 (2016): 176–99.
6 Kazakhstan was incorporated into the Kirghiz Autonomous Socialist Soviet Republic (1920–36), which included the territories of present-day Kazakhstan. It was renamed to Kazakh Soviet Socialist Republic in 1936.
7 Paula Michaels, *Curative Powers: Medicine and Empire in Stalin's Central Asia* (Pittsburgh: University of Pittsburgh Press, 2003).

8 A proper Soviet citizen was a class-conscious member of society who embodied the ethos of socialist modernity in which cleanliness, punctuality, trustworthiness, efficient work habits, and loyalty to the Soviet Communist Party sustained the well-ordered and centrally planned socialist economic machine. Nomadism stood in contradiction to proper Soviet conduct (see Tricia Starks, *The Body Soviet: Propaganda, Hygiene, and the Revolutionary State* [Madison: University of Wisconsin Press, 2008]).

9 Abigail Kret, "'We Unite with Knowledge': The Peoples' Friendship University and Soviet Education for the Third World," *Comparative Studies of South Asia, Africa, and the Middle East* 33, no. 2 (2013): 239–56; Olcott, *The Kazakhs*.

10 Isabelle Ohayon, *La Sédentarisation des Kazakhs dans l'URSS de Staline: Collectivisation et Changement Social (1928–1945)* (Paris: Maisonneuve et Larose-Institut Français d'études sur l'Asie Centrale, 2006); Isabelle Ohayon, "The Kazakh Famine: The Beginnings of Sedentarization," *SciencesPo: On-Line Encyclopedia of Mass Violence* (2013). https://www.sciencespo .fr/mass-violence-war-massacre-resistance/en/document/kazakh-famine -beginnings-sedentarization.html.

11 Douglas Northrop, *Veiled Empire: Gender and Power in Stalinist Central Asia* (Ithaca, NY: Cornell University Press, 2004); Lynne Viola, *Peasant Rebels Under Stalin: Collectivization and the Culture of Peasant Resistance* (Oxford: Oxford University Press, 1996). Historians Alter Litvin and John Keep (Alter Litvin and John Keep, *Stalinism: Russian and Western Views at the Turn of the Millennium* [London: Routledge, 2005], 58) suggest that in the thirty years between 1923 and Stalin's death in 1953, upwards of forty-one million people were convicted of various crimes like "work absenteeism" for not producing enough grain to meet (impossible) state mandated quotas or for "colluding with the enemy" (i.e., knowing someone whose political leanings were suspect). Millions of those individuals vanished into the vast archipelago of forced labour camps in Siberia and Central Asia, never to be heard from again (Aleksander Solzhenitsyn, *The Gulag Archipelago* [New York: Harper & Row, 1973]). Others were shot. Countless men, women, and children left behind starved to death in state-choreographed famines in Ukraine, the North Caucasus, and Kazakhstan. The scope and pace of Stalinist repressions were extraordinary: at the height of what historians refer to as the 1937–38 Great Terror campaign, over one and a third million people were arrested for various crimes and half of them were killed (Litvin and Keep, *Stalinism*). At that pace, the secret police executed on average 1867 individuals each day – 77 people per hour day and night (for one of the more powerful firsthand accounts of Stalin's terror see Eugenia Ginzburg, *Journey into the Whirlwind* [New York: Harcourt, Brace & World, 1967]). The recently opened KGB archives in Kazakhstan shed light

on the tragic chapter in Central Asia's history. Between the mid-1920s and 1956, millions of individuals died as a result of imprisonment, diseases, starvation, and executions. In 1937–38 alone, over twenty-five thousand members belonging to a Pan-Turkist movement among the elites in Kazakhstan were executed (Baktygul Chynybaeva, "Kazakhstan Opens Secret KGB Archives Amid Moves Toward Decolonization in Central Asia," *Radio Free Europe Radio Liberty*, November 12, 2023, 11:32 a.m. GMT, https://www.rferl.org/a/kazakhstan-opens-kgb-archives-russian-criticism/32681381.html).

12 Sarah Cameron, *The Hungry Steppe: Famine, Violence, and the Making of Soviet Kazakhstan* (Ithaca, NY: Cornell University Press, 2018); Niccolo Pianciola, "Famine in the Steppe: The Collectivization of Agriculture and the Kazakh Herdsmen, 1928–1944," *Cahiers du Monde Russe* 45, no. 1/2 (2004): 137–91; E.P. Zimovina, "Dinamika Chislennosti i Sostava Naseleniia Kazakhstana vo Vtoroi Polovine KhKh Veka" [Dynamics of the number and composition of the population of Kazakhstan in the second half of the 20th century], *Demoskop Weekly*, no. 103–104 (2003), http://www.demoscope.ru/weekly/2003/0103/analit03.php.

13 Karaganda Regional State Archive. f. 1487, op. 1. d. 84, l. 5.

14 *Spravochnik, Spravochnik po Istorii Kolkhozov, Sovkhozov i Drugikh Sel'skokhoziastvennykh Predpriiatii Karagandinskoi Oblasti* [Handbook, handbook of the history of Kolkhozes, Sovkhozes and other agricultural enterprises of the Karaganda region] (Karaganda, Kazakhstan: Odtel Arkhivov i Dokumentov Karagandinskoi Oblasti, 2012). 13.

15 *Spravochnik po Istorii* [Handbook of the history], 13.

16 *Spravochnik po Istorii* [Handbook of the history], 12.

17 All interviews are translated from the Russian by the author unless otherwise specified.

18 Khalid, "Backwardness and the Quest for Civilization: Early Soviet Central Asia in Comparative Perspective," 236.

19 See also Adeeb Khalid, *Central Asia: A New History from the Imperial Conquests to the Present* (Princeton, NJ: Princeton University Press, 2021).

20 See also Kate Brown, *Plutopia: Nuclear Families, Atomic Cities, and the Great Soviet and American Plutonium Disasters* (Oxford: Oxford University Press, 2013).

21 David Holloway, *Stalin and the Bomb: The Soviet Union and Atomic Energy, 1939–1956* (New Haven, CT: Yale University Press, 1994).

22 The Soviet Union conducted testing in two main areas: the southern Semipalatinsk Test Site and the northern Novaya Zemlya Arctic Archipelago (part of the Russian Federation) with a total energy yield equal to 285 megatons (Mt) of TNT, of which 247 Mt (or roughly 16,500 Hiroshima bombs) was released in above-ground detonations (V.N. Mikhailov, *Catalog of Worldwide Nuclear Testing* [New York: Ministry of Atomic Energy of the Russian Federation, Begell-Atom, 1999]). This equals a total of 742 nuclear tests with 969 charges

(Vitaly V. Adushkin and William Leith, *The Containment of Soviet Underground Nuclear Explosions, United States Geological Survey Open File Report 01-312* [Washington, DC: Department of the Interior Geological Survey, 2001], 6. On the Polygon, the test site and the military command centre were known by several other internal code-names, including Training Ground No. 2, *Ploshod M* (Site M), *Bereg* (riverbank), Semipalatinsk-21, and *Konechnaia* (ending or terminal) (S. Balmukhanov, G. Raissova, and T. Balmukhanov, *Three Generations of the Semipalatinsk Affected to the Radiation* (Almaty, Kazakhstan: Sakshy Press, 2002); Vadmim Logachev, ed., *Iadernye Ispytaniia SSSR. Semipalatinskii Poligon. Fakty, Svidetel'stva, Vospominaniia. Obespechenie Obsshchei i Radiatsionnoi Bezopasnosti Iadernykh Ispytanii* [Nuclear tests of the USSR. Semipalatinsk test site: Facts, evidence, memories. Ensuring general and radiation safety of nuclear tests] (Moscow, Russia: IGEM RAN, 1997), http://elib.biblioatom. ru/text/semipalatinskiy-poligon_1997/go,2/).

23 There is no agreement as to the total number of tests conducted on the Polygon, with the most-often-cited numbers varying between 527 and 456, depending on the source (Saim Balmukhanov, J. N. Abdrakhmanov, Timur Balmukhanov, Boris Gusev, Natalya Kurakina, and Tolegen Raisov, *Medical Effects and Dosimetric Data from Nuclear Tests at the Semipalatinsk Test Site: Technical Report* [Fort Belvoir, VA: Defense Threat Reduction Agency, 2006]; IAEA [International Atomic Energy Agency], *Radiological Conditions at the Semipalatinsk Test Site, Kazakhstan: Preliminary Assessment and Recommendations for Further Study. Radiological Assessment Reports Series 3* [Vienna: IAEA, 1998]). From my conversations with scientists conducting research in the region, most believe that the total number of all detonations (not just the number of tests that could have included the detonation of multiple bombs) is closer to 700. The number of charges is related to tests involving multiple nuclear devices detonated within milliseconds to seconds (known as salvo tests). Official sources report a total of 456 tests on the Polygon using 616 nuclear devices, with a total energy yield of 17.4 Mt of TNT (V.N. Mikhailov, ed., *USSR Nuclear Weapons Tests and Peaceful Nuclear Explosions, 1949 through 1990* [Moscow: Ministry of Atomic Energy and Ministry of Defense of the Russian Federation, 1996]). Within the Polygon, geographically diverse technical areas were selected for a range of nuclear tests. From 1949 to 1962, for example, testing was conducted on the Opytnoe Pole (Experimental Field, also known as site "P"). A total of 116 tests happened here above ground – either near the ground, in the atmosphere, or at high altitude. These tests were directed at weapons development and simulated nuclear war/combat engagements to collect data on the effects of blast, heat, and radioactive fallout on living organisms and machinery like planes, tanks, and other vehicles, as well as a host of structures like bridges and subway stations. Bombs were often dropped from planes and

platforms to analyse the impact of the blast. From 1949 to 1957, Soviet scientists conducted the most intense medical-biological experiments on mice, dogs, camels, and other animals (V.A. Logachev and L.A. Mikhalikhina, *Animal Effects from Soviet Atmospheric Nuclear Tests* (Fort Belvoir, VA: Defense Threat Reduction Agency, 2008), 6. Other testing areas include the Degelen Mountains, Sary-Uzen, Telkem, Balapan, Aktan-Berli, site 4, and site 4a, and other unnamed sites. The 4 and 4a technical areas were used to test radiological warfare agents manufactured from radiochemical waste, a fact that became known only in 2002 (Vakulchuk et al., *Semipalatinsk Nuclear Testing*). At the Degelen Mountain test field, 209 nuclear devices were exploded in horizontal tunnels (or adits, which have only one opening) that were drilled inside mountains, while diversion and damming of river experiments took place at the Balapan site (105 tests, including in boreholes). Sary-Uzen area saw twenty-four underground tests, some of which created the occasional crater and sometimes a retarc (an upside-down crater that looks like a mound). In 1963, the Limited Test Ban Treaty was signed by the United States, Great Britain, and the Soviet Union, prohibiting all nuclear tests in the atmosphere and underwater. Though the aims of the Limited Test Ban Treaty sought to reduce the spread of radioactive fallout, some of the subsequent underground explosions nevertheless vented radioactive particles into the atmosphere.

24 Nils-Olov Bergkvist and Ragnhild Ferm, *Nuclear Explosions 1945–1998* (Stockholm: Sipri Stockholm International Peace Research Institute; Defense Research Establishment Division of Systems and Underwater Technology, 2000).

25 Albert Baiburin, *The Soviet Passport: The History, Nature and Uses of the Internal Passport in the USSR* (Cambridge, UK: Polity Press, 2021); Lynne Viola, *The Unknown Gulag: The Lost World of Stalin's Special Settlements* (New York: Oxford University Press, 2007).

26 Edward Geist, *Armageddon Insurance: Civil Defense in the United States and Soviet Union, 1945–1991* (Chapel Hill: The University of North Carolina Press, 2019).

27 Two secret clinics were created in 1957 for systematic monitoring of the radiation situation and health status of residents of contaminated areas. Each had a clinical department, as well as biophysical and other laboratories. Dispensary No. 3, established in the city of Ust-Kamenogorsk, was disbanded in 1960 because of reduction in radioactive contamination of the area (Logachev, *Iadernye Ispytaniia SSSR* [Nuclear tests of the USSR]. Dispensary No. 4 operated under the pseudonym of Anti-Brucellosis Dispensary No. 4 of the USSR Ministry of Health from 1970.

28 Stanley Brunn, "Fifty Years of Soviet Nuclear Testing in Semipalatinsk, Kazakhstan: Juxtaposed Worlds of Blasts and Silences, Security and Risks,

Denials and Memory," in *Engineering Earth: The Impacts of Megaengineering Projects*, ed. Stanley Brunn (Dordrecht: Springer, 2011), 1789–818.

29 Logachev, *Iadernye Ispytaniia SSSR*; [Nuclear tests of the USSR] see also Susanne Bauer, "Beyond the Nuclear Epicenter: Health Research, Knowledge Infrastructures and Secrecy at Semipalatinsk," *Cahiers du Monde Russe* 60, no. 2–3 (2019): 493–516.

30 Aidar Atchabarov, "Kainar Syndrome: History of the First Epidemiological Case-Control Study of the Effects of Radiation and Malnutrition," *Central Asian Journal of Global Health* 4, no. 1 (2015): 221; Balmukhanov, et al., *Medical Effects*; Keshim Boztayev, *Sindrom Kainara* [Kainar syndrome] (Almaty, Kazakhstan: Atamura, 1994); Togzhan Kassenova, *Atomic Steppe: How Kazakhstan Gave Up the Bomb* (Stanford, CA: Stanford University Press, 2022); see also Brown, *Plutopia*.

31 "O Rabote Dispensera No4, za 1957 Jul-Dekabr," KGU Tsentr Dokumentatsii Noveyshey Istorii, f. 103, op. 73, d. 12, 3-12; Upravlenie Arkhivov i Dokumentatsii Vostochno-Kaxakhstankoi Oblasti. 2011. *Protivostoyaniye (Is Istorii Semipalatinskogo Politona). Sbornik Dodumentov.* Semey: KGU Tsentr Dokumentatsii Vostochno-Kazakhstanskoi Oblasti Nauchnyi Tsentr Istoricheskikh i Sotsial'no-Politicheskikh Issledovanii im. Adademika M. Kozybaeva Semipalatinskogo Gosudarstvennogo Pedagogicheskogo Instituta; V. Shepel' redaktor, otvet A. E. Abduali, A. E. Assanbaeva, E. M. Gribanova, Kazakhstan za Beziadernyi Mir. Sbornik Dokumentov i Materialov. Almaty: Arkhiv Presidenta Respubliki Kazakhstan. 2011 [On the work of Dispensary No4 for the year 1957 July-December, Center for Modern History Documentation of Eastern Kazakhstan, f. 103, op. 73, d. 12, 3-11; Department of Archives and Documentation of the East Kazakhstan Region. 2011. *Confrontation (from the history of the Semipalatinsk test site): A collection of documents.* Semey: Center for Modern History Documentation of Eastern Kazakhstan, The Academic M. Kozybayev Research Center for Historical and Socio-Political Studies of the Semipalatinsk State Pedagogical Institute; V. Shepel', eds., with A.E. Assanbaeva, E. M. Gribanova, contributors, Kazakhstan for a nuclear-free world: A collection of documents and materials. Almaty: Archive of the President of the Republic of Kazakhstan, 2011].

32 *Sindrom Kainara* [Kainar syndrome].

33 Martin McCauley, *Khrushchev and the Development of Soviet Agriculture: The Virgin Land Programme, 1953–1954* (New York, NY: Holmes and Meier, 1976).

34 Starks, *The Body Soviet.*

35 Marc Elie, "The Soviet Dust Bowl and the Canadian Erosion Experience in the New Lands of Kazakhstan, 1950s–1960s," *Global Environment* 8, no. 2 (2015): 259–92; see also Nikolai Dronin and Edward Bellinger, *Climate Dependence and Food Problems in Russia 1900–1990: The Interaction of Climate and Agricultural Policy and Their Effect on Food Problems* (Budapest: Central

European University Press, 2005); Paul Josephson, Nicolai Dronin, Ruben Mnatsakanian, Aleh Cherp, Dmitry Efremenko, and Vladislav Larin, eds., *An Environmental History of Russia* (Cambridge: Cambridge University Press, 2013); McCauley, *Khrushchev and the Development of Soviet Agriculture*; Zauresh Saktaganova, *Sovetskaia Modernizatsiia Ekonomiki Kazakhstana v 1946–70 gg: Kritika Istorichiskogo Opyta* [Soviet modernization of Kazakhstan's economy in 1946–70: A critique of historical experience] (Karaganda,: Kazakhstan Glasir, 2012).

36 Martin, *Law and Custom in the Steppe*.

37 McCauley, *Khrushchev and the Development of Soviet Agriculture*.

38 Germans and other exiles were sent to villages in northern Kazakhstan during the Second World War and were forced to stay after Stalin's death to carry out the Virgin Lands campaign. Northern Kazakhstan was also a vast penal region with hundreds of thousands of prisoners (Steven Barnes, *Death and Redemption: The Gulag and the Shaping of Soviet Society* [Princeton, NJ: Princeton University Press, 2011]). All were engaged in forced labour. Some of the political prisoners who worked on the Virgin Lands came from Karlag, a labour camp complex in central steppe in which people extracted coal and other ores and worked in rangeland animal husbandry.

39 Michaela Pohl, "The 'Planet of One Hundred Languages': Ethnic Relation and Soviet Identity in the Virgin Lands," in *Peopling the Russian Periphery: Borderland Colonization in Eurasian History*, ed. Nicholas Breyfogle, Abby Schrader, and Willard Sunderland (London: Routledge, 2007), 238–61; Viola, *The Unknown Gulag*. Kazakhstan's environmental history has everything to do with the heavy industrialization and militarism of the Soviet period. Early key sectors were developed inside the Gulag (Main Camp Administration), a vast network of prisons, forced labour camps, and exile communities that spread out across the Soviet Union (Barnes, *Death and Redemption*; Kate Brown, "Gridded Lives: Why Kazakhstan and Montana are Nearly the Same Place," *The American Historical Review* 106, no. 1 (2001): 17–48; Viola, *The Unknown Gulag*). In the 1930s through to the Second World War, the number of camps expanded dramatically. In Kazakhstan, prisoners extracted uranium, oil and gas, copper, coal, gold, and other resources. They built railways, roads, canals, and industrial infrastructure, including secret towns for atomic weapons development (Holloway, *Stalin and the Bomb*). Soviet industrialization and militarism, often a business cloaked in secrecy, led to the dumping of hundreds of millions of tons of toxins into the environment – this is of course, not unique to Kazakhstan or the former Soviet Union; the United States has a similar history (Andy Bruno, *The Nature of Soviet Power: An Arctic Environmental History* [Cambridge, UK: Cambridge University Press, 2016]; Brown, *Plutopia*; Mike Davis, *Dead Cities and Other Tales* [New York: The New Press, 2002]; Hugh Gusterson, *Nuclear Rites: A Weapons*

Laboratory at the End of the Cold War [Berkeley: University of California Press, 1996]; Barbara Rose Johnston, ed., *Half-Lives and Half-Truths: Confronting the Radioactive Legacies of the Cold War* [Santa Fe, NM: School for Advanced Research Press, 2007]; Josephson et al., *An Environmental History of Russia*; Valerie Kuletz, *The Tainted Desert: Environmental Ruin in the American West* [New York: Routledge, 1998]; Joseph Masco, 2006 *The Nuclear Borderlands: The Manhattan Project in Post–Cold War New Mexico* [Princeton, NJ: Princeton University Press, 2006]; Traci Voyles, *Wastelanding: Legacies of Uranium Mining in Navajo Country* [Minneapolis: University of Minnesota Press, 2015]). Rapid industrialization, coupled with scant public documentation and the cost of clean-up meant that monitoring and enforcing environmental standards was nearly impossible.

40 Pohl, "The 'Planet of One Hundred Languages,'" 238–61; Michaela Pohl, "From White Grave to Tselinograd to Astana: The Virgin Lands Opening, Khrushchev's Forgotten First Reform" in *The Thaw: Soviet Society and Culture during the 1950s and 1960s*, ed. Denis Kozlov and Eleonory Gilburd (Toronto: University of Toronto Press, 2013), 269–307.

41 "Ob Organizatsii v Kubskom Raionie Zernovykh Sovkhozov Karagandinskogo Gostresta Sovkhozov" [On the Organization of Grain State Farms in the Kubskii District under the Karaganda State Trust of State Farms], 1954, Karaganda Regional State Archive, f. 18, op. 1, d. 2061, l. 231–33; "O Vnesenii Imenii v Administrativno-terirtorial'noe Delenie Nekotorykh Sel'skikh Sovetov Deputatov Trudiashchikhsia Kubskogo Raiona" [On making changes to the administrative-territorial division of certain rural Council of Workers' Deputies], 1961, Karaganda Regional State Archive, f. 18 op. 1 d. 3309 l. 49.

42 The delaying of the end of the harvest by weeks or even months was a huge problem for agriculture in the Virgin Lands, especially acute in remote corners like Koian, where technical means to extract grain and ship it to silos were not good enough to do at the right agricultural time. This resulted in vast losses of grain. Nevertheless, even ineffective farming techniques still brought about social and cultural changes seen as positive by residents.

43 Murray Feshbach and Alfred Friendly, Jr., *Ecocide in the USSR: Health and Nature Under Siege* (New York: Basic Books, 1992); see also Paul Josephson, "Industrial Deserts: Industry, Science and the Destruction of Nature in the Soviet Union," *The Slavonic and East European Review* 85, no. 2 (2007): 294–321; Josephson et al., *An Environmental History of Russia*.

44 Elie, "The Soviet Dust Bowl and the Canadian Erosion Experience in the New Lands of Kazakhstan, 1950s–1960s," 259–92.

45 Zhanna Mazhitova, Aigul Zhalmurzina, Sveta Koganatova, Aitzhan Orazbakov, and Tastanbek Satbai, "Environmental Consequences of Khrushchev's Virgin Land Campaign in Kazakhstan (1950s–1960s)," *E3S Web of Conferences* 285, no. 05036 (2021): 1–12, https://www.e3s-conferences.

org/articles/e3sconf/abs/2021/34/e3sconf_uesf2021_05036/e3sconf_
uesf2021_05036.html.

46 Although beginning in the mid-1980s, ethnic Kazakhs demanded greater
freedom and autonomy in the decision-making processes within the Kazakh Soviet Socialist Republic, there was no official calls to secede from the
Soviet Union. Kazakhstan reluctantly declared independence on December
16, 1991, ten days before the formal dissolution of the Soviet Union.

47 Michael Burawoy and Katherine Verdery, eds., *Uncertain Transition: Ethnographies of Change in the Postsocialist World* (Lanham, MD: Rowman &
Littlefield, 1999); Susan Gal and Gail Kligman, *The Politics of Gender after
Socialism: A Comparative-Historical Essay* (Princeton, NJ: Princeton University Press, 2000); Bruce Grant, *In the Soviet House of Culture: A Century
of Perestroikas* (Princeton, NJ: Princeton University Press, 1995); Caroline
Humphrey, *The Unmaking of the Soviet Life: Everyday Economies after Socialism* (Ithaca, NY: Cornell University Press, 2002); Gail Kligman, *The Politics
of Duplicity: Controlling Reproduction in Ceausescu's Romania* (Berkeley: University of California Press, 1998); Joma Nazpary, *Post-Soviet Chaos: Violence
and Dispossession in Kazakhstan* (London: Pluto Press, 2002).

48 Catherine Alexander, "Value, Relations, and Changing Bodies: Privatization
and Property Rights in Kazakhstan" in *Property in Question: Value Transformation in the Global Economy*, ed. Caroline Humphrey and Katherine Verdery
(London: Routledge, 2004), 253; see also Nazpary, *Post-Soviet Chaos*.

49 There was an in-migration, too, when new national borders were redrawn
(Reeves, *Border Work*). Following independence, Kazakhstani state openly
encouraged ethnic Kazakhs (known as Oralman, meaning returnees) living in former Soviet republics, as well as in Mongolia and China to come
back. In 1997, several Kazakh Oralman families settled in Koian but left
after only a couple of years.

50 Agency on Statistics of the Republic of Kazakhstan, *Results of the 2009 National Population Census of the Republic of Kazakhstan: Analytical Report* (Astana, Kazakhstan: Agency on Statistics of the Republic of Kazakhstan, 2011).

51 It is worth noting that official statistics pertaining to the demographic
structure of Kazakhstan, although reflective of general trends, are nearly
useless in terms of reflecting the number of people living in any given
area. For example, Oktiabr' was listed as having nearly nine hundred people living in the village as of 2012, when in reality the number was closer
to 380. This discrepancy is a result of how people register their domicile
status, with those moving to the cities choosing to remain registered as living in the village to avoid paying municipal taxes and/or meeting specific
criteria, such as having a permanent job and place to live.

52 Electricity was shut off in the early 1990s and not turned back on until
2003. Villagers used kerosene lamps at night and would often describe this
period as *adskaia zhizn'* (hellish life).

53 See Astrid Mignon Kirchhof and John R. McNeill, eds., *Nature and the Iron Curtain: Environmental Policy and Social Movements in Communist and Capitalist Countries 1945–1990* (Pittsburgh, PA: Pittsburgh University Press, 2019).

54 Leila Hennaoui and Marzhan Nurzhan, "Dealing with a Nuclear Past: Revisiting the Cases of Algeria and Kazakhstan through a Decolonial Lens," *The International Spectator* 58, no. 4 (2023): 91–109; Hoover Institution Archives, Kazakh Subject Collection. Box 1 and Box 2 (see also Foreign Broadcast Information Service, *JPRS Report: Environmental Issues* (Springfield, VA: U.S. Department of Commerce National Technical Information Service, 1990); Melanie Arndt and Laurent Coumel, "A Green End to the Red Empire? Ecological Mobilizations in the Soviet Union and Its Successor States, 1950–2000: A Decentralized Approach," *Ab Imperio* 1 (2019): 105–24.

55 Kassenova, *Atomic Steppe*.

56 Sheila Fitzpatrick, *Everyday Stalinism: Ordinary Life in Extraordinary Times. Soviet Russia in the 1930s* (Oxford: Oxford University Press, 1999); see also Stephen Kotkin, *Magnetic Mountain: Stalinism as a Civilization* (Berkeley: University of California Press, 1997)

57 Donna M. Goldstein and Kira Hall, "Mass Hysteria in Le Roy, New York: How Brain Experts Materialized Truth and Outscienced Environmental Inquiry," *American Ethnologist* 42, no. 4 (2015): 640–57.

58 One aspect of "toxic layering" are the dust storms that carry aerosols that pose a threat to humans as they settle in lungs, wells, rivers, gardens, and livestock. When pesticides and radioactive elements are added to the mix, the dust can be deadly and very hard to trace back to one source.

59 Feshbach and Friendly, Jr., *Ecocide in the USSR*; Josephson et al., *An Environmental History of Russia*; According to anthropologist William Wheeler, Aral Sea communities also refuse to accept the narratives of environmental ruin as they undermine local pride (Wheeler, *Environment and Post-Soviet Transformation in Kazakhstan's Aral Sea Region*).

60 Laurent Coumel and Marc Elie, "A Belated and Tragic Ecological Revolution: Nature, Disasters, and Green Activists in the Soviet Union and the Post-Soviet States, 1960s–2010," *The Soviet and Post-Soviet Review* 40 (2013): 161.

61 Beginning in 1944, the order of "Mother Heroine" was given to women who had ten or more children. For raising a large family, the women were given financial assistance and increased food rations, and were able to collect higher pensions earlier than women with fewer children.

62 Svetlana Boym, *The Future of Nostalgia* (New York: Basic Books, 2001); Serguei Oushakine, "'We're Nostalgic but We're Not Crazy': Retrofitting the Past in Russia," *The Russian Review* 66, no. 3 (2007): 451–82.

63 Boris Gusev, Zhibek Abylkassimova, and Kazbek Apsalikov. "The Semipalatinsk Nuclear Test Site: A First Assessment of the Radiological Situation and the Test-Related Radiation Doses in the Surrounding Territories," *Radiation and Environmental Biophysics* 36, no. 3 (1997): 201–204.

64 Pohl, "The 'Planet of One Hundred Languages.'"
65 At the Polygon, while the numbers are imprecise, some medical doctors estimate that countless thousands of people were routinely exposed to radioactive fallout without ever knowing it, and many developed cancers as a result (B. Gusev, R. Rosenson, and Z. Abylkassimova, "The Semipalatinsk Nuclear Test Site: A First Analysis of Solid Cancer Incidence (Selected Sites) Due to Test-Related Radiation," *Radiation and Environmental Biophysics* 37, no. 3 (1998): 209–14). Although authorities gathered detailed scientific data on nuclear testing and how radiation effects plants, animals, and people since the mid-1950s, with the end of the Soviet Union, a great deal of data was removed from Kazakhstan and made inaccessible in Russia. A newly discovered report in the archives of the Institute of Radiation Medicine and Ecology in Semey, Kazakhstan recently revealed that several tests had severe impact on people. The August 12, 1953, thermonuclear device released 400 kilotons of TNT (or the equivalent of 26 Hiroshima sized bombs); 1956 nuclear test (a 27 Kt bomb) sent more than six hundred people in Ust-Kamenogorsk, roughly two hundred miles (320 kilometres) away from the Polygon, to the hospital with radiation sickness (Wudan Yan, "The Nuclear Sins of the Soviet Union Live on in Kazakhstan," *Nature*, April 3, 2019, https://www.nature.com/articles/d41586-019 -01034-8; see also Fred Pearce, "Exposed: Soviet Cover-Up of Nuclear Fallout Worse than Chernobyl," *New Scientist*, March 20, 2017, https:// www.newscientist.com/article/2125202-exposed-soviet-cover-up-of -nuclear-fallout-worse-than-chernobyl/). What this report also revealed is that the Soviets not only knew about health effects but also concealed them by blaming illnesses on poor diets and zoonotic diseases.
66 Brown, *Plutopia*.
67 Sergei Abashin, *Sovetskii Kishlak: Mezhdu Kolonialismom in Modernizatsiei [Soviet Kishlak: Between colonialism and modernization]* (Moscow: Novoe Literaturnoe Obozrenie, 2015); Kelly McMann, "The Shrinking of the Welfare State: Central Asians' Assessments of Soviet and Post-Soviet Governance," in *Everyday Life in Central Asia: Past and Present*, ed. Jeff Sahadeo and Russell Zanca (Bloomington, IN: Indiana University Press, 2007), 233–47.
68 Boym, *The Future of Nostalgia*, xiv; see also Laurent Coumel, Benjamin Guichard, and Walter Sperling, "Mémoires, Nostalgie et Usages Sociaux du Passé dans la Russie Contemporaine," *Le Mouvement Social* 260 (2017): 3–15; Lis Kayser, "Nuclear Nostalgia: Remembering the Nuclear Age on the Hao Atoll, French Polynesia" (PhD diss., University of Aarhus 2023); Lindsay A. Freeman, *Longing for the Bomb: Oak Ridge and Atomic Nostalgia* (Chapel Hill: The University of North Carolina Press, 2015). In Koian, people's narratives generally celebrate life in the sovkhoz. However, it could be argued that this celebration resembles the aesthetic ideal of what Milan Kundera

(1984) in *The Unbearable Lightness of Being* calls "Communist kitsch": "Kitsch excludes everything from its purview which is essentially unacceptable in human existence." In this formulation, the local representation of idyllic life on the Polygon during the time of the sovkhoz could be construed as a desperate attempt to affirm one's humanity or even, as "nuclear nostalgia" (Kayser, "Nuclear Nostalgia") – a way to hide and internalize what is intolerable in life and the violence that always lurked behind the idyllic every day. Yet this interpretation simply flies in the face of the fact that life was better in the sovkhoz than what came before or after.

69 In 1997, the Space Research Institute of the Ministry of Science and Education of the Republic of Kazakhstan found a massive 7700-square-mile (20,000-square-kilometre) thermal anomaly on the Polygon (U.M. Sultangazin, E.A. Zakharin, L.F. Spivak, O.P. Arhipkin, N.R. Muratova, A.G. Terehov, "Distantsionnoe Zondirovanie Temperaturnykh Anomalii v Raione Semipalatinskogo Iadernogo Poligona" [Remote sensing of thermal anomalies at the territory of the Semipalatinsk test site] *Lectures of Ministry of Science of the Academy of Science of the Republic of Kazakhstan* 6, no. 2 (1997): 51–4). During winter and spring, they noticed areas where snow either melted early or was entirely missing. The temperatures there were more than fifty degrees Fahrenheit (ten degrees Celsius) higher than the surrounding snowy areas, and almost no plants grew there during the growing season. The anomaly follows radioactive contamination of the Polygon. Some research suggests that it might be due to the ground heating up from hot fluids rising from deep underground fault zones, triggered by numerous nuclear explosions (Aleksander E. Velikanov, "About the Nature of Regional Thermal Anomaly in Semipalatinsk Test Site Region," *Mathematics and Computers in Simulation* 67, no. 4–5 [2004]: 459–65). Other research suggests that the anomaly is caused by the energy released from radioactive decay of certain elements left in the soil after surface and air explosions (Velikanov, "About the Nature of Regional Thermal Anomaly in Semipalatinsk Test Site Region"; see also Edige Zakarin, Larissa Balakay, Bibigul Mirkarimova, Natalia Tuseeva, Konstantin Pak, Alexander Baklanovm, Alexander Mahura, Jens H. Sorensen, *Geoinformation Modeling of Radionuclide Transfer from the Territory of the Semipalatinsk Test Site: FP6 EC CA – Enviro-RISKS: Man-Induced Environmental Risks: Monitoring, Management and Radiation of Man-made Changes in Siberia* (Copenhagen: Danish Meteorological Institute, 2008).

70 Walter Benjamin, "On the Concept of History," in *Selected Writings Volume 4: 1938–1940*, ed. Howard Eiland and Michael W. Jennings (Cambridge, MA: Harvard University Press, 2003), 392.

71 Michel Trouillot, *Silencing the Past: Power and the Production of History* (Boston, MA: Beacon Press, 1995).

Chapter 2

1 NNC (National Nuclear Center of the Republic of Kazakhstan, Institute of Radiation Safety and Ecology), *Semipalatinskii Ispytatel'nyi Poligon. Sovremennoe Sostoianie* [Semipalatinsk test site. Current state]. (Pavlodar, Kazakhstan: Press House, 2017), 16.

2 Johnston, ed., *Half-Lives and Half-Truths*.

3 Jonathan Metzl and Anna Kirkland, eds., *Against Health: How Health Became the New Morality* (New York: New York University Press, 2010).

4 Werner and Purvis-Roberts, "Cold War Memories and Post–Cold War Realities," 285–309; see also Per Hōgselius and Achim Klüpperlberg, *The Soviet Nuclear Archipelago: A Historical Geography of Atomic-Powered Communism* (Budapest: Central European University Press, 2024).

5 Petryna, *Life Exposed*.

6 Rob Nixon, *Slow Violence and the Environmentalism of the Poor* (Cambridge, MA: Harvard University Press, 2011).

7 Petryna, *Life Exposed*.

8 Robert Jacobs, *Nuclear Bodies: The Global Hibakusha* (New Haven, CT: Yale University Press, 2022.). Scientists in Semey who have spent their lives studying the biological aftermath of nuclear testing offered this observation: "One thing to remember, and this is very important, I think is that any radioecological disaster is unique. Japan is unique, our situation [at the Polygon] is also unique, Chornobyl is unique, Fukushima is unique. Chronic exposure is present in very few places around the world." See also Becky Alexis-Martin, *Disarming Doomsday: The Human Impact of Nuclear Weapons Since Hiroshima* (London: Pluto Press, 2019).

9 William Morgan and William Bair, "Issues in Low Dose Radiation Biology: The Controversy Continues. A Perspective," *Radiation Research* 179, no. 5 (2013): 501–10.

10 Tina Carlsen, Leif E. Peterson, Brant A. Ulsh, Cynthia A. Werner, Kathleen L. Purvis, and Anna C. Sharber, "Radionuclide Contamination at Kazakhstan's Semipalatinsk Test Site: Implications on Human and Ecological Health," *Human and Ecological Risk Assessment* 7, no. 4 (2001): 943–55.

11 S. Lochlann Jain, *Malignant: How Cancer Becomes Us* (Berkeley: University of California Press, 2013), 4, 14.

12 Donna Goldstein, "Experimentalité: Pharmaceutical Insights into Anthropology's Epistemologically Fractured Self," in *Medicine and the Politics of Knowledge*, ed. Susan Levine (Cape Town: HSRC Press, 2012), 119–52.

13 Adriana Petryna, *When Experiments Travel: Clinical Trials and the Global Search for Human Subjects* (Princeton, NJ: Princeton University Press, 2009).

14 NRC (National Research Council), *Health Risks from Exposure to Low Levels of Ionizing Radiation: BEIR VII, Phase 2* (Washington, DC: National Academies Press, 2006).

15 Biologist Timothy Mousseau, who is an expert on the effects of ionizing radiation on organisms living in Chornobyl (Chernobyl), Fukushima, and other radioactive regions around the world, disagrees. He argues that, in fact, there is no evidence to suggest that humans are more radioresistant than other mammals (Anders Møller and Timothy Mousseau, "Strong Effects of Ionizing Radiation from Chernobyl on Mutation Rates," *Scientific Reports* 5 [2015]: 8363, https://doi.org/10.1038/srep0863). Mousseau does suggest there is good evidence of genetically based differences among different species in how they show genetic damage in response to radiation, and there is abundant evidence to suggest that radiation can cause damage to the germ line (Hans Ellegren, Gabriella Lindgren, Craig Primmer, and Anders Pape Møller, "Fitness Loss and Germline Mutations in Barn Swallows Breeding in Chernobyl," *Nature* 389 [1997]: 593–96; Anders Møller, J. Erritzøe, F. Karadas, and Timothy Mousseau, "Historical Mutation Rates Predict Susceptibility to Radiation in Chernobyl Birds," *Journal of Evolutionary Biology* 23, no. 10 [2010]: 2132–42.). However, the data for humans are ambiguous (H. Weinberg, A. Korol, V. Kirzhner, A. Avivi, T. Fahima, E. Nevo, S. Shapiro, G. Rennert, O. Piatek, E. Stepanova, and E. Skvarskaja, "Very High Mutation Rate in Offspring of Chernobyl Accident Liquidators," *Proceedings of the Royal Society B* 268, no. 1471 [2001]: 1471–2954; Meredith Yeager et al. "Lack of Transgenerational Effects of Ionizing Radiation Exposure from Chernobyl Accident," *Science* 375, no. 6543 [2021]: 725–29).
16 NRC (United States Nuclear Regulatory Commission) "Backgrounder on Biological Effects of Radiation," *United States Nuclear Regulatory Commission* (2015), https://www.nrc.gov/reading-rm/doc-collections/fact-sheets/bio-effects-radiation.html.
17 Nixon, *Slow Violence and the Environmentalism of the Poor.*
18 Balmukhanov et al., *Three Generations of the Semipalatinsk Affected to the Radiation*; Bauer et al., "Radiation Exposure Due to Local Fallout from Soviet Atmospheric Nuclear Weapons Testing in Kazakhstan"; Bernd Grosche, "Semipalatinsk Test Site: Introduction," *Radiation and Environmental Biophysics* 41, no. 1 (2002): 53–55; Z. Zhumadilov, B. Gusev, J. Takada, M. Hoshi, A. Kimura, N. Hayakawa, and N. Takeichi, "Thyroid Abnormality Trend Over Time in Northeastern Regions of Kazakstan, Adjacent to the Semipalatinsk Nuclear Test Site: A Case Review of Pathological Findings for 7271 Patients," *Journal of Radiation Research* 41 (2000): 35–44.
19 Vakulchuk et al., *Semipalatinsk Nuclear Testing.*
20 "Genetic Effects of Radiation in the Offspring of Atomic-Bomb Survivors," Radiation Effects Research Foundation, accessed February 15, 2015, https://www.rerf.or.jp/en/programs/roadmap_e/health_effects-en/geneefx-en/
21 Charles Perrow, "Nuclear Denial: From Hiroshima to Fukushima," *Bulletin of the Atomic Scientists* 69, no. 5 (2013): 56–67.

22 Gayle Greene, *The Woman Who Knew Too Much: Alice Stewart and the Secrets of Radiation* (Ann Arbor: University of Michigan Press, 1999); Gayle Greene, "Science with a Skew: The Nuclear Power Industry after Chernobyl and Fukushima," *The Asia-Pacific Journal* 10, no. 1 (2012): 3.

23 Goldstein and Stawkowski, "James V. Neel and Yuri E. Dubrova," 67–98; see also Brown, *Plutopia*; Angela Creager, *Life Atomic: A History of Radioisotopes in Science and Medicine* (Chicago, IL: University of Chicago Press, 2013); Samuel J. Walker, "The Atomic Energy Commission and the Politics of Radiation Protection, 1967–1971," *Isis* 85, no. 1 (1994): 57–78.

24 M.I. Balonov, "Review of 'Chernobyl: Consequences of the Catastrophe for People and the Environment,' by Alexey V. Yablokov, Vassily B. Nesterenko, and Alexey V. Nesterenko," *Annals of the New York Academy of Sciences* 1181 (December 2009), http://www.nyas.org/asset.axd?id =8b4c4bfc-3b35-434f-8a5c-ee5579d11dbb&t=634507382459270000; James Neel, "Two Recent Radiation-Related Genetic False Alarms: Leukemia in West Cumbria, England, and Minisatellite Mutations in Belarus," *Teratology* 59, no. 4 (1999): 302–306.

25 Yuri Dubrova, Valeri N. Nesterov, Nicolay G. Krouchinsky, Vladislav A. Ostapenko, Rita Neumann, David L. Neil, and Alec J. Jeffreys, "Human Minisatellite Mutation Rate after the Chernobyl Accident," *Nature* 380, no. 6576 (1996): 683–86.

26 Brown, *Plutopia*.

27 Brown, *Plutopia*.

28 William DeJong-Lambert, *The Cold War Politics of Genetic Research: An Introduction to the Lysenko Affair* (Dordrecht: Springer, 2012).

29 NNC (National Nuclear Center of the Republic of Kazakhstan, Institute of Radiation Safety and Ecology), *Semipalatinsk Nuclear Test Site: Present State.* (Pavlodar, Kazakhstan: Press House, 2011), 46.

30 NNC, *Semipalatinsk Nuclear Test Site*, 46.

31 IAEA, *Radiological Conditions at the Semipalatinsk Test Site, Kazakhstan*; NNC, *Semipalatinsk Nuclear Test Site*, 46.

32 For example, Milana Guzeeva, "Nevidimye Miru Dozy" [Doses invisible to the world], *Vremya*, April 27, 2013, http://www.time.kz/articles/risk /2013/04/27/nevidimie-miru-dozi.

33 Catherine Alexander, "Nettoyer et Tourner la Page: La Renaissance Nucléaire du Kazakhstan" [Cleaning up and moving on: Kazakhstan's nuclear renaissance], in *Les Chantiers du Nucléaire*, ed. Romain Garcier and Françoise Lafaye (Paris: Archives Contemporaines, 2016), 3.

34 Alexander, "Cleaning Up and Moving On: Kazakhstan's Nuclear Renaissance," 3.

35 Alexander, "Cleaning Up and Moving On: Kazakhstan's Nuclear Renaissance," 4.

36 K. Kadyrzhanov and S. Lukashenko, "Radioactivity in Kazakhstan. Cases and Consequences," in *Environmental Protection Against Radioactive Pollution*, ed. Nevzat Birsen and Kairat Kadyrzhanov (Dordrecht, Netherlands: Kluwer Academic Publishers, 2003), 11–18; see also NNC (National Nuclear Center), Republic of Kazakhstan Institute of Radiation Safety and Ecology, *Institute of Radiation Safety and Ecology* (Pavlodar, Kazakhstan: Press House, 2012).

37 Psychological stress has been used to explain illness claims long before Chornobyl (Chernobyl). One of the earliest mentions of radiophobia I found is by a French physician and gynecologist, François Foveau de Courmelles, who defined it as an irrational and paranoid fear of X-rays (François Foveau de Courmelles, "Radiophobia," *The Lancet* 16 [1935]: 1153). Although not explicitly defined as radiophobia, psychological stress was also observed in the Hiroshima and Nagasaki atomic bomb survivors and in populations who lived through the Three Mile Island nuclear power plant accident in Pennsylvania, among others (Daniel L., Collins, Andrew Baum, and Jerome E. Singer, "Coping with Chronic Stress at Three Mile Island: Psychological and Biochemical Evidence," *Health Psychology* 2, no. 2 (1983): 149–66; Robert Lifton, *Death in Life: Survivors of Hiroshima* [Chapel Hill: University of North Carolina Press, 1991]).

38 Evelyn Bromet, "Mental Health Consequences of the Chernobyl Disaster," *Journal of Radiological Protection* 32, no. 1 (2012): 71–75; R. Perez Foster, D. Branovan, and G. Ukrainsky, *Surviving Chernobyl in America: Medical and Mental Health Consequences of the Chernobyl Nuclear Accident* (New York: Media Luna Ltd, 2003); IAEA, *One Decade after Chernobyl: Summing Up the Consequences of the Accident: Proceedings of an International Conference on One Decade After Chernobyl: Summing Up the Consequences of the Accident* (Vienna: IAEA, 1996); L. Ilyin and O. Pavlovskij. "Radiological Consequences of the Chernobyl Accident in the Soviet Union and Measures Taken to Mitigate their Impact," *IAEA Bulletin* 4 (1987): 17–24; Z. Jaworowski, "Observations on Chernobyl After 25 Years of Radiophobia," *21st Century Science & Technology* (Summer 2010): 30–45; A. Rumyantsev, "Remarks by the Minister of the Russian Federation for Atomic Energy," in *Security of Radioactive Sources*, ed. IAEA (Vienna: IAEA, 2003), 15–18; I. Yevelson, A. Abdelgani, J. Cwikel, and I. Yevelson, "Bridging the Gap in Mental Health Approaches between East and West: The Psychosocial Consequences of Radiation Exposure," *Environmental Health Perspectives* 105, suppl. 6 (1997), 1551–56.

39 Chernobyl Forum, *Chernobyl's Legacy: Health, Environmental and Socio-Economic Impacts and Recommendations to the Governments of Belarus, the Russian Federation and Ukraine* (Vienna: IAEA, 2005).

40 Edward Schatz, "Notes on the 'Dog That Didn't Bark': Eco-Internationalism in Late Soviet Kazakhstan," *Ethnic and Racial Studies Review* 22, no. 2

(1999), 136–61; Kassenova, *Atomic Steppe;* Werner and Purvis-Roberts, "After the Cold War," 461–80; Werner and Purvis-Roberts, "Cold War Memories and Post–Cold War Realities," 285–309. Qualification for these benefits is based on risk estimates of past radiation exposure. Despite its proximity to the Polygon, Koian is considered a zone of minimal radiation risk, and most Koianers received a one-time payment of about fifty dollars.

41 "Home page," the ATOM Project, http://www.theatomproject.org/en/.

42 Werner and Purvis-Roberts, "After the Cold War," 461–80.

43 Timothy Mousseau and Sarah Todd, "Biological Consequences of Exposure to Radioactive Hydrogen (Tritium): A Comprehensive Survey of the Literature," *SSRN* (2023), https://papers.ssrn.com/sol3/papers.cfm?abstract_id=4416674; Lyubov Timonova et al., "Tritium Distribution in the 'Water-Soil-Air' System in the Semipalatinsk Test Site," *PLoS ONE* 19, no. 4 (2024): e0297017, https://doi.org/10.1371/journal.pone.0297017.

44 NNC, *Semipalatinskii Ispytatel'nyi Poligon* [Semipalatinsk test site], 12.

45 Cindy Folkers, "Fukushima Catastrophe at 6: Normalizing Radiation Exposure Demeans Women and Kids and Risks Their Health," *Counter Punch*, March 6, 2017, http://www.counterpunch.org/2017/03/06/fukushima-catastrophe-at-6-normalizing-radiation-exposure-demeans-women-and-kids-and-risks-their-health/.

46 See also Gregory Button, *Disaster Culture: Knowledge and Uncertainty in the Wake of Human and Environmental Catastrophe* (Walnut Creek, CA: Left Coast Press, 2010).

47 David Harvey, *The Condition of Postmodernity* (Cambridge, UK: Blackwell, 1990).

48 Henry Giroux, "Reading Hurricane Katrina: Race, Class, and the Biopolitics of Disposability," *College Literature* 33, no. 3 (2006), 171–96.

49 Didier Fassin, *When Bodies Remember: Experiences and Politics of AIDS in South Africa* (Berkeley: University of California Press, 2007), 115.

50 Brown, *Manual for Survival*; see also Svetlana Alexievich, *Voices from Chernobyl: The Oral History of a Nuclear Disaster* (New York: Picador, 2006); Rosalie Bertell, "Chernobyl: An Unbelievable Failure to Help," *International Journal of Health Services* 38, no. 3 (2008): 543–60; Leon Gouré, *The Medical Aspects of the Chernobyl Nuclear Reactor Accident, Draft Report. Prepared for the Defense Nuclear Agency and OSD/Net Assessment. Leon Gouré Papers, Box 15.7. Hoover Institution Archives* (Stanford, CA: Stanford University Press, 1987); Olga Kuchinskaya, *The Politics of Invisibility: Public Knowledge about Radiation Health Effects after Chernobyl* (Cambridge, MA: MIT Press, 2014); Serhii Plokhy, *Chernobyl: The Hisotry of a Nuclear Catastrophe* (New York: Basic Books, 2018); Wladimir Wertelecki, "Malformations in a Chernobyl-Impacted Region," *Pediatrics* 125, no. 4 (2010): e836–e843.

51 Greene, *The Woman Who Knew Too Much.*

52 Several studies on the psychological effects of nuclear testing have been conducted in the Polygon region (N. Kawano, K. Hirabayashi, M. Motsuo, Y. Taooka, T. Hiraoka, K. Apsalikov, T. Moldagaliev, and M. Hoshi, "Human Suffering Effects of Nuclear Tests at Semipalatinsk, Kazakhstan: Established On the Basis of Questionnaire Surveys," *Journal of Radiation Research* 47, suppl, (2006): A209–A217; G. Jumazhanova, G. Tursungozhinova, O. Belenko, M. Iskakova, and A. Amanova, "Ecological Consciousness of a Personality Living in an Ecologically Unfavorable Region," *International Journal of Environmental and Science Education* 11, no. 7 (2016): 1469–78; K. Purvis-Roberts, C. Werner, and I. Frank, "Perceived Risks from Radiation and Nuclear Testing Near Semipalatinsk, Kazakhstan: A Comparison Between Physicians, Scientists, and the Public," *Risk Analysis* 27, no. 2 (2007): 291–302). These were based on questionnaire surveys that gathered information from people living in and around the site, as well as from scientists and physicians working in the region. The studies generally conclude that the higher perceptions of risk among local populations, compared to those of professionals, are, in part, due to lack of scientific knowledge about radiation risk (see also Wynne's discussion of the "public deficit" model of scientific understanding in Brian Wynne, *Rationality and Ritual: Participation and Exclusion in Nuclear-Decision Making* [London: Earthscan, 2011]). Regarding internal exposure, one study concluded that although the site is contaminated with significant amounts of "bone-seeking" strontium-90, "countermeasures to protect the population from enhanced radiation exposure at the [Polygon] are currently not necessary, provided the inhabitants are warned about some very localized hot spots that should be fenced to restrict entry by humans or grazing animals" (N. Semioshkina and G. Voigt, "An Overview on GSF Activities at the Semipalatinsk Test Site, Kazakhstan," *Journal of Radiation Research* 47, suppl. [2006]: A98; see also Vadim Logachev, L.A. Mikhalikhina, Natalya Darenskaya, A. Matuschchenko, Yuri Stepanov, and O. Shamov, *Population Health in Regions Adjacent to the Semipalatinsk Nuclear Test Site. AFRRI Contract Report 98-94* [Bethesda, MD: Armed Forces Radiobiology Research Institute, 1998]).

53 Susanne Bauer, "Tracing Mutations: Biodosimetry Tools in Post–Cold War Radiation Epidemiology," in *Making Mutations: Objects, Practices, Contexts*, ed. Luis Campos and Alexander von Schwerin (Berlin: Max Planck Institute for the History of Science, 2010), 209.

54 Dubrova et al., "Human Minisatellite Mutation Rate after the Chernobyl Accident," 683–86; Yuri Dubrova, Rakhmet I. Bersimbaev, Leila B. Djansugurova, Maira K. Tankimanova, Zaure Zh. Mamyrbaeva, Riitta Mustonen, Carita Lindholm, Maj Hultén, and Sisko Salomaa, "Nuclear Weapons Tests and Human Germline Mutation Rate," *Science* 295, no. 5557 (2002): 1037.

55 Nori Nakamura, "Genetic Effects of Radiation in Atomic-Bomb Survivors and Their Children: Past, Present and Future," *Journal of Radiation Research* 47, suppl. B (2006): B67–B73.

56 "Current Threat," the ATOM Project, accessed February 10, 2015, http://www.theatomproject.org/en/current-threat.

57 Antony Butts, *After the Apocalypse* (London: Tigerlily Films, 2010), DVD.

58 Troy Duster, *Backdoor to Eugenics* (New York: Routledge, 1990).

59 Agamben, *Homo Sacer*.

60 Nancy Scheper-Hughes, "Mr. Tati's Holiday and João's Safari – Seeing the World through Transplant Tourism," *Body and Society* 17, no. 2–3 (2011): 55–92.

61 Didier Fassin, *Humanitarian Reason: A Moral History of the Present* (Berkeley: University of California Press, 2012).

62 Sherry Ortner, "Subjectivity and Cultural Critique," *Anthropological Theory* 5, no. 1 (2005): 31–52.

63 There was one person with a mental disability, a man born with webbed feet, a woman with one slightly short thumb, and several people with vitiligo, but serious and life-threatening deformities were nowhere to be found.

64 Petryna, *Life Exposed*.

65 Otto Binder, "How Nuclear Radiation Can Change Our Race," *Mechanix Illustrated*, December 1953, 109.

66 Heather Paxson, *The Life of Cheese: Crafting Food and Value in America* (Berkeley: University of California Press, 2012).

67 Donna Haraway, *When Species Meet* (Minneapolis: University of Minnesota Press, 2008).

68 CTBTO (Comprehensive Nuclear-Test-Ban Treaty Organization), *On-Site Inspections: The Ultimate Verification Measure* (Vienna: Preparatory Commission for the CTBTO, 2009), 1, 2.

69 "CTBTO Inspectors Implement On-Site Inspection Test Scenario in Kazakh Steppe," CTBTO, accessed March 3, 2015, http://www.ctbto.org/press-centre/highlights/2008/ctbto-inspectors-implement-on-site-inspection-test-scenario-in-kazakh-steppe.

70 Sarah Phillips, "Half-Lives and Healthy Bodies: Discourses on 'Contaminated' Food and Healing in Post-Chernobyl Ukraine," *Food & Foodways* 10 (2002): 27–53.

71 Anders Møller and Timothy Mousseau, "The Effects of Low-Dose Radiation: Soviet Science, the Nuclear Industry – and Independence?" *Significance* 10, no. 1 (2013): 14–19; see also Timothy Mousseau and Anders Møller, "Genetic and Ecological Studies of Animals in Chernobyl and Fukushima," *Journal of Heredity* 105, no. 5 (2014): 704–709.

72 Joseph Masco, "Mutant Ecologies: Radioactive Life in Post–Cold War New Mexico," *Cultural Anthropology* 19, no. 4 (2004): 518; see also Paul Rabinow, "Artificiality and Enlightenment: From Sociobiology to Biosociality," in

Essays on the Anthropology of Reason (Princeton, NJ: Princeton University Press, 1996), 91–111.

73 Gilles Deleuze and Félix Guattari, *A Thousand Plateaus: Capitalism and Schizophrenia*, trans. Brian Massumi (Minneapolis: University of Minnesota Press, 1987).

74 Masco, "Mutant Ecologies," 517–50.

Chapter 3

1 It took more than a decade for the villagers to rebuild their herds. Some families did better than others. The poorest might have three cows, one horse, and fifteen sheep. Others like Tursynbek were better off, having six horses, about thirty cows, and over fifty sheep and goats. In comparison, I visited a singular prosperous family that lived an hour's drive away in a zimovka, and was told they owned 320 cows, 250 horses, and 1200 sheep and goats. According to Livestock Summary Report for Oktiabr', in 2010, Koian had 262 cows, 972 sheep, 904 goats, and 435 horses in total. Oktiabr' had 1783 cows, 6996 sheep, 1212 goats, and 416 horses. The Report also lists 70 poultry in Koian, although I did not see any chickens, geese, or other birds in the village.

2 Antoine Volodine (2017) wrote a superb novel and political commentary in *Radiant Terminus*. The book is a story about a postapocalyptic dystopian future in the wake of nuclear meltdowns and the fall of the second Soviet Union. In the novel, Volodine examines camps as spaces of mutual aid and fatalistic brotherhood because the camp is a place where individuals come together in times of crisis to support one another. Much like residents of Volodine's camp, Koian residents are bound together by their shared struggles and experiences, the village functioning as a self-contained system in which survival is possible only through mutual support. Despite the hardships, Koianers are comforted by their collective endeavours, which foster a sense of solidarity. This sense of solidarity, as I show in this chapter, is a response to the vast inequalities exacerbated by the post-Soviet economic transformations.

3 Humphrey, *The Unmaking of the Soviet Life*, 75; see also James Ferguson, *Give a Man a Fish: Reflections on the New Politics of Distribution* (Durham, NC: Duke University Press, 2015).

4 Judith Butler, *Frames of War: When Is Life Grieivable?* (New York: Verso, 2009), 14.

5 James Ferguson and Tania Murray Li, *Beyond the 'Proper Job:' Political-economic Analysis after the Century of Labouring Man, Working Paper 51* (Cape Town: PLAAS, UWC, 2018); see also ILO (International Labour Organization), *World Employment and Social Outlook: Trends 2018* (Geneva: International Labour Office, 2018); Jean Comaroff and John Comaroff, "After Labor," *Critical Historical Studies* 7, no. 1 (2020): 87–112.

6 Michael Denning, "Wageless Life," *New Left Review* 66 (2010): 79–97.

7 Ian Shaw and Marv Waterstone, *Wageless Life: A Manifesto for a Future beyond Capitalism* (Minneapolis: University of Minnesota Press, 2019), 78. It should be noted that the majority of people around the world do not and never will work in traditional wage jobs (what would be considered full-time salaried employment). Today, among those who are employed worldwide, more than half are in temporary, part-time, on-call, or dependent self-employment with falling wages (ILO [International Labour Organization], *World Employment and Social Outlook: Trends 2022* [Geneva: International Labour Office, 2022]. Insecurity has dominated labour for most of human existence (Jan Breman, "A Bogus Concept?" *New Left Review* 84 [2013]: 130–38; Jan Breman, "A Short History of the Informal Economy," *Global Labour Journal* 14, no. 1 [2023]: 21–39; Ferguson, *Give a Man a Fish*; Ronaldo Munck, "The Precariat: A View from the South," *Third World Quarterly* 34, no. 5 [2013]: 747–62).

8 Denning, "Wageless Life," 79–97; see also Chris Hann and Jonathan Parry, eds., *Industrial Labor on the Margins of Capitalism: Precarity, Class, and the Neoliberal Subject* (New York: Berghahn, 2018); Carolina Humphrey and David Sneath, *The End of Nomadism? Society, State and the Environment in Inner Asia* (Durham, NC: Duke University Press, 1999); Sian Lazar and Andrew Sanchez, "Understanding Labor Politics in an Age of Precarity," *Dialectical Anthropology* 43, no. 1 (2019): 3–14; Rebecca Prentice, "Work after Precarity: Anthropologies of Labor and Wageless Life," *Focaal – Journal of Global and Historical Anthropology* 88 (2020): 117–24.

9 Kathleen Millar, *Reclaiming the Discarded: Life and Labor on Rio's Garbage Dump* (Durham, NC: Duke University Press, 2018), 8. In her ethnography of garbage pickers (*catadores*) working the vast landfill on the outskirts of Rio de Janeiro, Millar argues for decentring wage work. Her account shows that for the dump workers, wage labour is undesirable and they prefer scavenging the landfill that has become a source of income, autonomy, and a "good life."

10 MDG (Millennium Development Goals) Report, *Millennium Development Goals in Kazakhstan* (New York: United Nations Development Programme, 2010); United Nations, *United Nations in Kazakhstan Annual Report 2021* (Geneva: United Nations, 2021). These goals are as follows: (1) eradicate extreme poverty and hunger; (2) achieve universal primary education; (3) promote gender equality and empower women; (4) reduce child mortality; (5) improve maternal health; (6) combat HIV/AIDS, malaria, and other diseases; (7) ensure environmental sustainability; and (8) create a global partnership for development (https://www.un.org/millenniumgoals/).

11 World Bank, *Macro Poverty Outlook: Kazakhstan* (Washington, DC: World Bank, 2022), https://thedocs.worldbank.org/en/doc/d5f32ef28464d01

f195827b7e020a3e8-0500022021/related/mpo-kaz.pdf. In 2022, 58 percent of the country's GDP came from oil (https://www.trade.gov /country-commercial-guides/kazakhstan-market-overview). As a result, Kazakhstan's economy is susceptible to sharp economic upturns and downturns. Since 2000, Kazakhstan's economy has been growing at an annual rate of eight percent, making it one of the ten fastest-growing economies in the world (OECD [Organisation for Economic Co-operation and Development], *Multi-dimensional Review of Kazakhstan. Volume 1. Initial Assessment* [Paris: OECD Publishing, 2016]; OECD, *Multi-dimensional Review of Kazakhstan: Volume 2. In-Depth Analysis and Recommendations* [Paris: OECD Publishing, 2017]). The growth of the economy slowed significantly with the COVID-19 pandemic.

12 World Bank Group, *World Bank Group-Kazakhstan Partnership Program Snapshot* (Astana, Kazakhstan: World Bank, 2015); see also World Bank Group, *Doing Business 2020: Comparing Business Regulation in 190 Economies* (Washington, DC: International Bank for Reconstruction and Development/The World Bank, 2020).

13 Hilary Appel and Mitchell Orenstein, "Why did Neoliberalism Triumph and Endure in the Post-Communist World?" *Comparative Politics* 48, no. 3 (2016): 313–31; Nazpary, *Post-Soviet Chaos*; Katherine Verdery, *What Was Socialism, and What Comes Next?* (Princeton, NJ: Princeton University Press, 1996).

14 Saipira Furstenberg, "Applying a Global Governance Agenda in Post-Soviet States: The Case of EITI in Kazakhstan and Kyrgyzstan" (PhD diss., University of Exeter, 2017); David Harvey, "Neoliberalism as Creative Destruction," *The Annals of the American Academy of Political and Social Science* 610 (2007): 22–44.

15 Barbara Junisbai, "A Tale of Two Kazakhstans: Sources of Political Cleavage and Conflict in the Post-Soviet Period," *Europe-Asia Studies* 62, no. 2 (2010): 235–69.

16 Pauline Jones-Luong and Erika Weinthal, *Oil Is Not a Curse: Ownership Structure and Institutions in Soviet Successor States* (New York: Cambridge University Press, 2010).

17 Saulesh Yessenova, "The Tengiz Oil Enclave: Labor, Business, and the State," *Polar* 35, no. 1 (2012): 94–114.

18 Sherry Ortner, "On Neoliberalism," *Anthropology of this Century*, 1 (May 2011), http://aotcpress.com/articles/neoliberalism/.

19 Before 1991, subsidies for agriculture were 12 per cent of the GDP. In 1993, this number was around 2 per cent of the GDP, and between 1995 and 1999 subsidies for agriculture were virtually nonexistent (Martin Petrick and Richard Pomfret, "Agricultural Policies in Kazakhstan," IAMO Discussion Papers no. 155 [Leibniz Institute of Agricultural Development in Transition Economies, 2016]).

20 OECD (The Organisation for Economic Co-operation and Development), *OECD Review of Agricultural Policies: Kazakhstan 2013* (Paris: OECD Publishing, 2013).

21 Daniel Hayward, "Kazakhstan-Context and Land Governance," *Land Portal* (June 23, 2022), https://landportal.org/book/narratives/2022/kazakhstan#ref16; Vasyl Kvartiuk and Martin Petrick, "Liberal Land Reform in Kazakhstan? The Effect on Land Rental and Credit Markets," *World Development* 138 (2021): 105285; Ministry of Justice of the Republic of Kazakhstan, *Land Code of the Republic of Kazakhstan. Code of the Republic of Kazakhstan Dated 20 June, 2003, No. 442* [in Russian] (Astana, Kazakhstan: Legal Information System of Regulatory Legal Acts of the Republic of Kazakhstan, 2003), https://adilet.zan.kz/eng/docs/K030000442_. The original Land Code allowed for ninety-nine-year leases. The Code was amended in 2001 to forty-nine years.

22 Petrick and Pomfret, "Agricultural Policies in Kazakhstan"; Carole Ferret, "Mobile Pastoralism a Century Apart: Continuity and Change in South-Eastern Kazakhstan, 1910 and 2012," *Central Asian Survey* 37, no. 4 (2018): 503–25. The number of cattle fell from nine million to less than four million (Petrick and Pomfret, "Agricultural Policies in Kazakhstan"). With collapse across all sectors of the economy, people returned to their villages or used the garden plots attached to their country houses to become self-sufficient (Petrick and Pomfret, "Agricultural Policies in Kazakhstan").

23 Kvartiuk and Petrick, "Liberal Land Reform in Kazakhstan?," 105285.

24 As of 2019, only 1.4 per cent of Kazakhstan's agricultural land is privately owned, and leasing is the predominant way people access it (Kvartiuk and Petrick, "Liberal Land Reform in Kazakhstan?," 105285). Kazakhstan's vertical structure of authority means that its president appoints governors to the seventeen regions of Kazakhstan, with each governor appointing district akims (local executive leaders), who have extensive authority over land rights (Margaret Hanson, "Legalized Rent-Seeking: Eminent Domain in Kazakhstan," *Cornell International Law Journal* 50, no. 1 [2017]: 15–46). Until 2021, district akims appointed the next-level akims, all the way down to the village level. President Kassym-Jomart Tokaev's reform in 2021 allowed people to directly choose local leadership.

25 According to the villagers, a person from the capital Astana leased land for livestock breeding near Koian. He made use of workers (mostly from Uzbekistan) that he kept in slavery-like conditions. These workers, whose passports were taken, received housing and food in exchange for their labour. Stories about labour slavery are common in Kazakhstan. For example, in 2012, a resident of Karaganda spent more than one year in slave labour before he was rescued (Elena, Veber, "Zhitelia Karagandy Neskol'ko Raz Pereprodavali v Rabstvo" [A resident of Karaganda was resold into

slavery several times], *Radio Azattyk*, March 29, 2012, https://rus.azattyq.
org/a/rabstvo_vladimir_temirtau_tarabukina_/24530747.html). In 2014,
five people around Koian escaped from a winter farm, with one person
having spent twelve years in abysmal conditions (Dana Mendybaeva,
"Zhiteli Karagandinskoi Oblasti Bezhali iz Rabstva" [Residents of Karaganda region escaped from slavery], *Novyi Vestnik*, March 1, 2014, http://
nv.kz/2014/03/01/67620/).

26 Iliya Alimaev and Roy Behnke, "Ideology, Land Tenure and Livestock
Mobility in Kazakhstan," in *Fragmentation in Semi-Arid and Arid Landscapes*,
ed. Kathleen A. Galvin, Robin S. Reid, Roy H. Behnke Jr., and N. Thompson
Hobbs (London: Springer Nature, 2008), 151–78.

27 Alimaev and Behnke, "Ideology, Land Tenure and Livestock Mobility in
Kazakhstan," 151–78; Markus Hauck, Gulzhan Artykbaeva, Tamara Zozulya, and Choimaa Dalamsuren, "Pastoral Livestock Husbandry and Rural
Livelihoods in the Forest-Steppe of East Kazakhstan," *Journal of Arid Environments* 133 (2016): 102–11.

28 Alena Ledeneva, *Russia's Economy of Favors: Blat, Networking and Informal
Exchange* (London: Cambridge University Press, 1998); Alena Ledeneva,
*How Russia Really Works: The Informal Practices that Shaped Post-Soviet
Politics and Business* (Ithaca, NY: Cornell University Press, 2006); Edward
Schatz, *Modern Clan Politics: The Power of "Blood" in Kazakhstan and Beyond*
(Seattle: University of Washington Press, 2004); Rivkin-Fish, *Women's
Health in Post-Soviet Russia*; Charles Walker, "Space, Kinship Networks and
Youth Transition in Provincial Russia: Negotiating Urban-Rural and In-
ter-Regional Migration," *Europe-Asia Studies* 62, no. 4 (2010): 647–69; Abel
Polese, "What Is Informality? (Mapping) 'the Art of Bypassing the State' in
Eurasian Spaces – and Beyond," *Eurasian Geography and Economics* 64, no. 3
(2021): 322–64. Jeremy Morris and Abel Polese, eds., *The Informal Post-
Socialist Economy: Embedded Practices and Livelihoods* (London: Routledge,
2013); David Henig and Nicolette Makovicky, eds., *Economies of Favour
after Socialism* (Oxford: Oxford University Press, 2013). Jeremy Morris and
Abel Polese (*The Informal Post-Socialist Economy*) argue that it would be a
mistake to see "informal economies" as vestiges that corrupt and "institu-
tionally deficient" post-socialist societies are prone to. Informal economic
activities, understood as those unregulated by the state, including barter,
stealing, economy of favours, and so on (Verdery, *What Was Socialism,
and What Comes Next?*), are not only increasing but are also embedded in
the formal economic sector, sustained by the very structure of capitalism
and part and parcel of it (see also Rano Turaeva, "Informal Economies
in Post-Soviet Space: Post-Soviet Islam and Its Role in Ordering Entrepreneurship in Central Asia," *Central Asian Affairs* 5, no. 1 [2018]: 57–75).
The problematic classification of economies as "informal" and therefore

the "negative" by-product of scarcity is common in scholarly literature (Keith Hart, "Informal Income Opportunities and Urban Employment in Ghana," *The Journal of Modern African Studies* 11, no. 1 [1973]: 61–89; Keith Hart, "The Informal Economy," *The Cambridge Journal of Anthropology* 10, no. 2 [1985]: 54–58; Ulrich Beck, *The Brave New World of Work* [Cambridge, UK: Polity Press, 2000]; Zygmunt Bauman, *Wasted Lives: Modernity and Its Outcasts* [Cambridge, UK: Polity Press, 2004]); Mike Davis, *Planet of Slums* [London: Verso, 2006]). What is classified as informal is still debated in scholarly literature because the term includes such diverse activities as domestic work, gambling, mining, field tilling, street selling, begging, garbage collecting, and others that don't neatly fit into this category (Millar, *Reclaiming the Discarded*). Recent investigations around Chornobyl (Chernobyl) nuclear Exclusion Zone in Ukraine have shown an advent of "informal economies" in the region within the context of a retiring and retreating state that has abandoned its commitments to certain geographic areas (Thom Davies and Abel Polese, "Informality and Survival in Ukraine's Nuclear Landscape: Living with the Risks of Chernobyl," *Journal of Eurasian Studies* 6, no. 1 [2015]: 34–45).

29 Ferguson and Li, *Beyond the "Proper Job."*
30 Hart, "Informal Income Opportunities and Urban Employment in Ghana," 61–89; Polese, "What is Informality?," 322–64.
31 According to individuals I spoke to in the village, meat can be sold only in the oblast' (administrative region) of residence. Hence, even though the city of Semey is much closer to Koian than Karaganda, Koian residents cannot sell their meat products there.
32 The store owners in Oktiabr' claim that shuttling products from the city is expensive, and the cost of food and shuttling services simply reflect that. Furthermore, they also point out that most people who buy in their store do so on credit that they pay off whenever they are able.
33 Both brucellosis and *siberiiska iazva* (anthrax) are animal borne diseases and pose serious health risks to humans. Some individuals in Koian have had both at one point in their lives. While rarely fatal, they nevertheless cause fevers, severe joint and muscle pain, headaches, and fatigue – all of which can become chronic.
34 There is no state organization dedicated to measuring radiation levels in food products, including those coming from regions in and around the Polygon.
35 Tursynbek's cow that day sold for six dollars per kilogram. As he noted, he often was forced to sell a cow for as low as 700 USD, but according to colleagues living in Karaganda, the sale price for Tursynbek's cow was still too low. Between 2010 and 2012, food prices were relatively stable in Kazakhstan, and at the bazar prices were as follows: milk 150 Tenge/litre, a loaf of bread 60 Tenge, ground beef 1500 Tenge/kilogram, beef strips 2700

Tenge/kilogram, beer 250 Tenge/litre, and grilled lamb *shashlik* (a skewer of about five pieces of meat) 1000 Tenge. Sheep and goats from Koian were sold in Karaganda anywhere from 10,000 to 15,000 Tenge (or 68 to 102 USD, respectively).

36 During my 2010–11 fieldwork in Kazakhstan, one dollar equalled 147 Tenge on average. In 2015, the Tenge collapsed after the government took steps against supporting the currency. In 2019, one dollar was worth 334 Tenge on average.

37 In summer 2022, the cost of buying a sheep was about 40,000 Tenge (or 84 USD).

38 In recent years, various multinational mining ventures operate on the former test site with the permission of the National Nuclear Center of the Republic of Kazakhstan and hire local stockbreeders like Tursynbek to work in open pits – operations that seemed to change management each year. When I visited one such mine with Tursynbek, he wanted me to measure radioactivity in the area, but I wasn't allowed to do that (it turns out no one is allowed to measure radioactivity on their own – in fact my presence with a Geiger counter meant that Tursynbek was repeatedly questioned about it afterwards). His earnings from supplemental labours plus that of the rest of his extended family of seven in Koian were between 60,000 and 140,000 Tenge per month (400 and 950 USD).

39 Northrop, *Veiled Empire*; Cynthia Werner, "Bride Abduction in Post-Soviet Central Asia: Marking a Shift Towards Patriarchy through Local Discourses of Shame and Tradition," *The Journal of the Royal Anthropological Institute* 15, no. 2 (2009): 314–31.

40 Tatyana Mamonova, *Women's Glasnost vs. Naglost: Stopping Russian Backlash* (Westport, CT: Bergin and Garvey, 1994); Natalia Roudakova and Deborah Ballard-Reisch, "Femininity and the Double Burden: Dialogues on the Socialization of Russian Daughters into Womanhood," *Anthropology of East Europe Review* 17, no. 1 (1999): 21–34.

41 Deniz Kandiyoti, "The Politics of Gender and the Soviet Paradox: Neither Colonized, Nor Modern?," *Central Asian Survey* 26, no. 4 (2008): 601–23; Phyllis Moen, *Women's Two Roles: A Contemporary Dilemma* (Westport, CT: Auburn House, 1992).

42 Eva-Marie Dubuisson and Anna Genina, "Claiming an Ancestral Homeland: Kazakh Pilgrimage and Migration in Inner Asia," *Central Asian Survey* 30, no. 3–4 (2011): 469–85; Gal and Kligman, *The Politics of Gender after Socialism*; Aksana Ismailbekova, "Migration and Patrilineal Descent: The Role of Women in Kyrgyzstan," *Central Asian Survey* 33, no. 3 (2014): 375–89; Diana Kudaibergenova, "Between the State and the Artist: Representations of Femininity and Masculinity in the Formation of Ideas of the Nation in Central Asia," *Nationalities Papers* 44, no. 2 (2018): 225–46;

Mishtal, *The Politics of Morality*; Rivkin-Fish, *Women's Health in Post-Soviet Russia*; Azamat Sarsembaev, "Imagined Communities: Kazak Nationalism and Kazakification in the 1990s," *Central Asian Survey* 18 (1999): 319–46.

43 Judith Beyer and Peter Finke, "Practices of Traditionalization in Central Asia," *Central Asian Survey* 38, no. 3 (2019): 310–28; Kandiyoti, "The Politics of Gender and the Soviet Paradox," 601–23; Kathleen Kuehnast and Carol Nechemias, eds., *Post-Soviet Women Encountering Transition: Nation Building, Economic Survival, and Civic Activism* (Baltimore, MD: Johns Hopkins University Press, 2004); Anara Tabyshalieva, "Revival of Traditions in Post-Soviet Central Asia," in *Making the Transition Work for Women in Europe and Central Asia*, ed. Marnia Lazreg (Washington, DC: World Bank, 2000).

44 Éva Fodor, "Gender and the Experience of Poverty in Eastern Europe and Russia after 1989," *Communist and Post-Communist Studies* 35, no. 4 (2002): 369–82; Nanette Funk, "Feminist Critiques of Liberalism: Can They Travel East? Their Relevance in Eastern and Central Europe and the Former Soviet Union," *Signs* 29, no. 3 (2004): 695–726; Cynthia Werner, Christopher Edling, Charles Becker, Elena Kim, Russell Kleinbach, Fatima Esengeldievna Sartbay and Woden Teachout, "Bride Kidnapping in Post-Soviet Eurasia: A Roundtable Discussion," *Central Asian Survey* 37, no. 4 (2018): 582–601.

45 James Ferguson, *Expectations of Modernity: Myths and Meanings of Urban Life on the Zambian Copperbelt* (Berkeley: University of California Press, 1999).

46 Silvia Federici, *Caliban and the Witch: Women, the Body and Primitive Accumulation* (Brooklyn, NY: Autonomedia, 2018).

47 Werner, "Bride Abduction in Post-Soviet Central Asia," 314–31; Werner et al., "Bride Kidnapping in Post-Soviet Eurasia," 582–601. Bride abduction is not a traditional marriage practice in Kazakhstan and rarely occurred in the pre-Soviet period (Werner, "Bride Abduction in Post-Soviet Central Asia," 314–31). Most marriages were arranged by family members who sought to establish kinship ties. During the Soviet era, bride abduction was outlawed as a "crime of custom." Today, like before, the married couple cannot be related within seven generations (only on the male side) and the bride moves into her husband's family home.

48 Cynthia Werner, "Women, Marriage, and the Nation-State: The Rise of Nonconsensual Bride Kidnapping in Post-Soviet Kazakhstan," in *The Transformation of Central Asia: States and Societies from Soviet Rule to Independence*, ed. Pauline Jones-Luong (Ithaca, NY: Cornell University Press, 2004), 59–90; Werner, "Bride Abduction in Post-Soviet Central Asia," 314–31.

49 Werner, "Bride Abduction in Post-Soviet Central Asia," 314–31.

50 Diana Kudaibergenova, "Project Kelin: Marriage, Women, and Re-Traditionalization in Post-Soviet Kazakhstan," in *Women of Asia: Globalization, Development, and Gender Equity*, ed. Mehrangiz Najafizadeh and Linda Lindsey (New York: Routledge, 2018), 379–90.

51 Kudaibergenova, "Project Kelin," 381; Werner, "Women, Marriage, and the Nation-State," 59–90.

52 Although motherhood is celebrated in Kazakhstan as a moral duty, most women in Koian had two children only and most were on birth control in the form of an intrauterine device. Women accessed birth control at clinics. It was never made clear to me whether they accessed birth control in secret, without their husband's knowledge. Moreover, some women who were abducted (even with consent) left their husbands and moved back to their family home.

53 Junisbai, "A Tale of Two Kazakhstans," 235–69; Morgan Liu, *Under Solomon's Throne: Uzbek Visions of Renewal in Osh* (Pittsburgh, PA: University of Pittsburgh Press, 2012).

54 The lands of the Polygon belong to three regions: the Abai region (east Kazakhstan region until June 8, 2022), Pavlodar region, and Karaganda region. According to Semyon, the environmental activist I worked with in Karaganda, regional authorities have not issued a single permit for use of the Polygon lands for farming or livestock breeding, while the Abai (formerly east Kazakhstan) region at the time issued hundreds of such permits, including ones for collecting scrap metal. According to Semyon, in 2008, in the east Kazakhstan region alone, there were fifty-seven farms, where thirteen thousand sheep, six hundred horses and twenty-five hundred cows were kept. That year, some 145 tons of meat was produced in the region. Semyon believes that in 2022, the numbers of animals were much higher, although no one seems to keep track of the numbers of people who use the Polygon pastures.

55 Recently, the 2017 *Law on Pastoralism* was passed regarding the management of pastures, allowing district-level pasture use planning, which regulates access while looking to prevent land degradation. However, the Land Code also grants the *akimat* (local executive government) extensive authority over land rights, including the right to eminent domain (Hanson, "Legalized Rent-Seeking," 15–46).

56 Catherine Alexander, "Homeless in the Homeland: Housing Protests in Kazakhstan," *Critique of Anthropology* 38, no. 2 (2018): 204–20; Petryna, *Life Exposed*; Johnston and Barker, *Consequential Damages of Nuclear War*. Sociologist Javier Auyero and anthropologist Débora Alejandra Swistun (*Flammable*) observed something similar in an Argentine shantytown where residents doubt and deny harmful impact of pollution.

57 In March 2011, Burkut's youngest son (who was twenty-three years old at the time) went missing. When the local police refused to help find him, residents of surrounding villages began a search on their own. After three weeks of scouring the steppe, they located his body lying in a ditch beneath the snow. The police established the official cause of death as hypothermia, but I was told there was evidence of defensive wounds.

Chapter 4

1 Natalie Koch and Kristopher White, "Cowboys, Gangsters, and Rural Bumpkins: Constructing the 'Other' in Kazakhstan's 'Texas,'" in *Legitimacy, Symbols, and Social Changes*, ed. M. Laruelle (Lanham, MD: Lexington Books, 2016), 181–207.

2 see Nazym Shedenova and Aigul Beimisheva, "Social and Economic Status of Urban and Rural Households in Kazakhstan," *Procedia-Social and Behavioral Sciences* 82 (2013): 585–91.

3 Pierre Bourdieu, "The Forms of Capital," in *Handbook of Theory and Research for the Sociology of Education*, ed. John G. Richardson (New York: Greenwood Press, 1986), 241–58.

4 Donna M. Goldstein, *Laughter Out of Place: Race, Class, Violence, and Sexuality in a Rio Shantytown* (Berkeley: University of California Press, 2013 [2003]).

5 Saulesh Yessenova, "Routes and Roots of Kazakh Identity: Urban Migration in Postsocialist Kazakhstan," *Russian Review* 64, no. 4 (2005): 666.

6 Yessenova, "Routes and Roots of Kazakh Identity," 661–79; see also Alima Bissenova, "The Fortress and the Frontier: Mobility, Culture, and Class in Almaty and Astana," *Europe-Asia Studies* 69, no. 4 (2017): 642–67; Bhavna Davé, *Kazakhstan: Ethnicity, Language and Power* (New York: Routledge, 2007); Natalie Koch, "Bordering on the Modern: Power, Practice and Exclusion in Astana," *Transactions* 39, no. 3 (2013): 432–43; Mateusz Laszczkowski, *City of the Future: Building Space, Modernity, and Urban Change in Astana* (New York: Berghahn, 2016); Nazpary, *Post-Soviet Chaos*; Giulia Panicciari, "Almaty as a New Kazakh City: Kazakhisation of Urban Spaces after Independence," in *Changing Urban Landscapes: Eastern European and Post-Soviet Cities since 1989*, ed. M. Buttino (Rome: Viella, 2012); Saulesh Yessenova, *The Politics and Poetics of the Nation: Urban Narratives of Kazakh Identity* (Saarbrücken, Germany: LAP Lambert Academic Publishing, 2010).

7 Koch and White, "Cowboys, Gangsters, and Rural Bumpkins," 181–207.

8 Raymond Williams, *The Country and the City* (London: Chatto and Windus, 1973).

9 Yessenova, *The Politics and Poetics of the Nation.*

10 There are two terms to explain here as they refer to villagers on the Polygon. As I understood their usage, both are extremely derogatory. *Poligonskie* denotes any person who lives or has lived near the test site and likely carries the meaning that there is something abnormal, genetically mutated, or polluted about them. *Bogatye*, while in Russian meaning "wealthy," in this case seemed to suggest "thief," "cheater," "squatter," or "bandit." On occasion when I heard bogatye, it was assumed that villagers performed a certain level of poverty, especially in appearance, to disguise their wealth.

11 Khrushchëvki are low-cost and drab three- to five-storey housing blocks
with dozens of small apartments made of brick or concrete panels. They
were named after Soviet leader Nikita Khrushchev who sought to resolve
a post–World War II housing crisis and overcrowding in cities. The residential buildings offer little in terms of comfort: no elevators, insulation,
or living space. In Kazakhstan, many of these apartment blocks are in
disrepair.

12 Ian Hacking, "Making People Up," in *Reconstructing Individualism: Auton-
omy, Individuality, and the Self in Western Thought*, ed. Thomas C. Heller,
Morton Sosna, and David E. Wellbery (Stanford, CA: Stanford University
Press, 1986), pp. 222–36; Nancy Scheper-Hughes, *Saints, Scholars, and Schiz-
ophrenics: Mental Illness in Rural Ireland* (Berkeley: University of California
Press, 1982).

13 In their work on Kazakhstan's nation-building project, anthropologists
Eva-Marie Dubuisson and Anna Genina ("Claiming an Ancestral Homeland," 470) argue that "rootedness and movement are not antithetical but
rather co-present in the experience of a Kazakh homeland as a cyclical
inhabitation of landscape and ancestry." They observe that the ways in
which people organize their sense of belonging is informed by different
social, political, economic, and historical contexts and do not necessarily
correspond to the borders of the nation-state.

14 McGranahan, "Theorizing Refusal," 319–25; Audra Simpson, "On Ethnographic Refusal: Indigeneity, 'Voice' and Colonial Citizenship," *Junctures* 9
(2007): 67–80; Audra Simpson, *Mohawk Interruptus: Political Life Across the
Borders of Settler States* (Durham, NC: Duke University Press, 2014); Audra
Simpson, "Consent's Revenge," *Cultural Anthropology* 31, no. 3 (2016): 326–33.

15 McGranahan, "Theorizing Refusal," 319.

16 Simpson, "On Ethnographic Refusal," 78.

17 McGranahan, "Theorizing Refusal," 320.

18 Anthropologists and other scholars have sought to explain and understand acts of resistance in various social, political, economic, and historical
contexts (Ranajit Guha, *Elementary Aspects of Peasant Insurgency in Colonial
India* [Delhi: Oxford University Press, 1983]; Aihwa Ong, *Spirits of Resistance and Capitalist Discipline: Factory Women in Malaysia* [Albany: State University of New York Press, 1987]; Michael Taussig, *The Devil and Commodity
Fetishism in South America* [Chapel Hill: University of North Carolina Press,
1980]; James Scott, *Weapons of the Weak: Everyday Forms of Peasant Resistance*
[New Haven, CT: Yale University Press, 1985]). At the same time, the term
is notoriously difficult to define, and anthropologists have reflected on
what acts count and don't count as resistance (Lila Abu-Lughod, "The Romance of Resistance: Tracing Transformations of Power Through Bedouin
Women," *American Ethnologist* 17, no. 1 [1990]: 41–55; Sherry Ortner,

"Resistance and the Problem of Ethnographic Refusal," *Comparative Studies in Society and History* 37, no. 1 [1995]:173–93; Nancy Scheper-Hughes, "The Primacy of the Ethical: Propositions for a Militant Anthropology," *Current Anthropology* 36, no. 3 [1995]: 409–40). Refusal is not just another word for resistance but rather a way to stake a claim in the level of engagement to participate in (McGranahan, "Theorizing Refusal).

19 With the unravelling of the Soviet Union, scientists, and in this particular case, biologists, who once relied on the government for employment, found their laboratories either severely underfunded or found themselves without a job altogether. As research funding dwindled, many looked across borders to foreign biologists for assistance. Beginning in 1993, international European organizations like INTAS provided an economic lifeline and in the process stemmed a serious brain drain from the newly independent post-Soviet states like Kazakhstan. An influx of money meant that collaborative research projects between local and foreign scientists were sought after commodities. For local and international scientists, the once secret Soviet era Semipalatinsk Test Site – closed in 1991 at the behest of Kazakhstan President Nursultan Nazarbaev – presented itself as a radiobioecological laboratory. Some local officials I talked to encouraged this view, referring to the Polygon as a "perfect natural laboratory inhabited by people." They cast the uniqueness of the Polygon as an opportunity to study long-term radiobiological processes in plants and animals, as well as to assess genetic damage in people. These same local officials also envisioned the international community as a source of income to the entire region, which had suffered dramatic economic decline after the end of the Cold War.

20 From 1990 to 2019, cancer and cardiovascular disease were the two leading causes of death in Kazakhstan (Gabriel Gulis, Altyn Aringazina, Zhamilya Sangilbayeva, Kalel Zhan, Evelyne de Leeuw, and John Allegrante, "Population Health Status of the Republic of Kazakhstan: Trends and Implications for Public Health Policy," *International Journal of Environmental Research and Public Health* 18 (2021): 12235. In the Koian region, children were more than nine times likely to develop digestive system diseases, 1.4 times more likely to develop skin diseases, and eight times more likely to develop chronic genitourinary (relating to genital and urinary organs) diseases than a control group (in addition to blood pathologies, mental and behavioural disorders, respiratory system disorders, congenital anomalies, and other pathologies) (Almagul Kuzgibekova, Gulmira Muldayeva, Bibigul Abeuova, Galina Yeryomicheva, Dinagul Baesheva, Venara Tashkenbayeva, Aigul Takirova, Bibigul Tukbekova, Meiram Askarov, and Kamshat Zhumakanova, "The State of Health of Children Living in Adverse Environmental Conditions," *Australasian Medical*

Journal 9, no. 12 [2016]: 474–80; see also Akbaya Markabaeva, Susanne Bauer, Ludmila Pivina, Geir Bjorklund, Salvatore Chirumbolo, Aiman Kerimkulova, Yuliya Semenova, and Tatyana Belikhina, "Increased Prevalence of Essential Hypertension in Areas Previously Exposed to Fallout Due to Nuclear Weapons Testing at the Semipalatinsk Test Site, Kazakhstan," *Environmental Research* 167 [2018]: 129–35; Yuliya Semenova, Ludmila Pivina, Almira Manatova, Geir Bjorklund, Natalya Glushkova, Tatyana Belikhina, Marzhan Dauletyarova, and Tamara Zhunussova, "Mental Distress in the Rural Kazakhstani Population Exposed and Non-Exposed to Radiation from the Semipalatinsk Nuclear Test Site," *Journal of Environmental Radioactivity* 203 [2019]: 39–47). Moreover, high rates of anaemia, cardiovascular diseases (in one town of about two thousand people, 32 per cent of the adult population), and cancers occur (M. Aliyakparov, N. Kozachenko, A. Abisheva, R. Dosmagambetova, and I. Galstrev, *Mediko-Ekologicheskie Problemy Karagandinskogo Regiona: Populiatsionnye Issledovaniia Poslednego Desiatiletiia* [Medical and ecological problems of the Karaganda region: Population studies of the last decade] [Karaganda, Kazakhstan: Agenstvo Respubliki Kazakhstan po Delam Zdravookhraneniia, 2001]; Yuna Korostelyova, "Regional Pathology: How Long-Term Nuclear Weapons Tests Have Affected the Health of People Living Nearby" [in Russian] [n.d.], https://polygon.vlast.kz/health). Kazakhstan's Ministry of Health has called cancer an oncological crisis. Over the past twenty years, the incidence of cancer has increased by 25 per cent, even though mortality has decreased by 33 per cent ("In Kazakhstan, Over the Past 20 Years, Mortality from Cancer Has Decreased by 33%," Prime Minister of the Republic of Kazakhstan, accessed March 5, 2024, https://primeminister.kz/ru/news/v-kazakhstane-za-poslednie-20-let -smertnost-ot-onkologicheskikh-zabolevaniy-snizilas-na-33-23189). Incidence rates in the northeastern regions (the area of the Polygon) exceed the national figures by 1.5 times. Breast cancer, lung cancer, and stomach cancer (in that order) are most frequent. There is no complete set of data on how radiation impacts human health. The studies on the impact of the Polygon are scattered and focus only on certain aspects or places. In addition, some data that should be available are missing altogether, much of it hauled away to Russia after the fall of the Soviet Union and inaccessible to researchers. The latest report from the Institute of Public Policy and Administration at the University of Central Asia tries to tackle this by looking at all the health impacts related to nuclear testing on the Polygon. The report found "exceptionally large consequences for a wide range of health conditions many decades after the explosions ceased" (Charles Becker, Jeffery Hill, and Sultan Muratov, "Brighter than a Million Suns: Contemporary Health Consequences of Atomic Testing in the

Semipalatinsk Nuclear Polygon." IPPA Working Paper Series: Working Paper #70 [Bishkek, Kyrgyzstan: University of Central Asia, 2022, 1]).

21 Vanessa Agard-Jones, "Bodies in the System," *Small Axe* 17, no. 3 (42) (2013): 182–92.

22 Bauer, "Tracing Mutations," 209.

23 Nickolas Rose, *The Politics of Life Itself: Biomedicine, Power, and Subjectivity in the Twenty-First Century* (Princeton, NJ: Princeton University Press, 2006).

24 Rose, *The Politics of Life Itself.*

25 Susanne Bauer, "Radiation Science After the Cold War. The Politics of Measurement, Risk and Compensation in Kazakhstan," in *Health, Technologies, and Politics in Post-Soviet Settings: Navigating Uncertainties,* ed. Olga Zvonareva, Evgeniya Popova, and Klasien Horstman (Cham, Switzerland: Palgrave Macmillan, 2017), 225–49.

26 Tania Murray Li, *Land's End: Capitalist Relations on an Indigenous Frontier* (Durham, NC: Duke University Press, 2014).

27 Logachev, *Iadernye Ispytaniia SSSR* [Nuclear tests of the USSR] Some attempts at examinations of populations were carried out by military doctors between 1949 and 1953. These studies, however, were done without laboratory and clinical study designs, and documentation of findings was minimal. Essentially, the early studies were selective and largely random in nature (Logachev, *Iadernye Ispytaniia SSSR* [Nuclear tests of the USSR]. The situation changed with the first thermonuclear test in 1953, when a radioactive cloud travelled hundreds of kilometres beyond the Polygon. Major research expeditions took place between 1956 and 1960 under the direction of the Moscow Institute of Biophysics of the Soviet Union Academy of Medical Sciences, and between 1957 and 1959 by the Institute of Regional Pathology, Kazakh Academy of Sciences, under the direction of Bakiia Atchabarov (authorized by the President of the Academy of Sciences of the Kazakh SSR, Kanysh Satpaev) and Saim Balmukhanov, chief radiologist of the Ministry of Health of the Kazakh SSR, who conducted separate early investigations through their personal initiative. The Kazakh studies produced twelve volumes of reports. At a conference in Moscow in 1962, representatives of the Institute of Biophysics reported findings from their expeditions (they found minimal radiation impact), which were kept secret from Ministry of Health of the Kazakh SSR and the Academy of Sciences of the Kazakh SSR. They were opposed by Kazakh researchers from the Institute of Regional Pathology, who claimed that cumulative symptoms of residents of Semipalatinsk and nearby villages indicated radiation sickness. The leadership of the Kazakh SSR, which initially approved the expeditions, did not defend the positions of the researchers and followed instructions from Moscow, prohibiting further study of radioactive contamination (Bakiia Atchabarov, *Zablushdeniia, Lozh' i Istina po Voprosu Otsenki Vliianiia na Zdorov'e Liudei*

Ispytaniia Atomnogo Oruzhii na Semipalatinskom Iadernom Poligone [Misconceptions, lies and truths on the issue of assessing the health impact of nuclear weapons testing at the Semipalatinsk nuclear test site] [Almaty, Kazakhstan: Karzhy-Karazhat, 2002]; Saim Balmukhanov, *The Semipalatinsk Nuclear Test Site – Through My Own Eyes* [Fort Belvoir, VA: Defense Technical Information Center, 2014]). In total, there were six expeditions to the region between 1956 and 1960: 1956, 1957, 1958, 1959, and 1960 (Logachev 1997). In 1960, a cohort of twenty thousand exposed (experimental) and unexposed (control) village inhabitants was established and followed longitudinally. Congenital malformations, cancers, and other health issues were regularly reported. The available archives reflect that widespread radioactive contamination of milk, carrots, grain, apples, as well as meat at the Semipalatinsk meat plant, among other food products in the latter part of 1965 often exceeded norms by as much as sixty times (A.A. Aubakirov et al., *Protivsostoyaniye (Iz Istorii Semipalatinskogo Poligona). Sbornik Dokumentov* [Confrontation (from the history of the Semipalatinsk test site): A collection of documents] [Semey, Kazakhstan: Upravlenie Arkhivov *i* Dokumentatsii Vostochno-Kazakhstanskoi Oblasti, 2011], 29, 31–34. The level of contamination was never shared with the public, and meat that was marked for export was consumed instead locally. On September 10, 1956, 272 troops landed near a nuclear test epicenter 43 minutes after the blast to access performance, but no data exists on the outcome (B. M. Botev, "Ministry of Defense in the Atomic Project," Atom 81 [2019]: 9–10). Despite some data collection, I was told by scientists working in Kurchatov that monitoring of radioactive fallout was uneven. For example, only twenty-four of the above-ground tests, most moving in the northeasterly direction (towards the cities of Kurchatov, Semipalatinsk, and Ust-Kamenogorsk), were tracked. The remainder of fallout was not precisely mapped and much of the data are not accessible. Very little information has been preserved about the organization of meteorological support for early nuclear tests, and the first Semipalatinsk meteorological training ground was created only in 1954 (V.N. Mikhailov, ed., *Iadernye Ispytaniia SSSR. Tom 2: Tekhnologii Iadernykh Ispytanii SSSR. Vozdeistvie na Okruzhaiushchuiu Sredu. Mery po Obespecheniiu Bezopasnosti. Iadernye Poligony i Ploshchadki* [Nuclear tests of the USSR. Volume 2: Nuclear technologies of USSR tests. Environmental impact. Security measures. Nuclear testing sites and platforms] [Sarov, Russia: RFYATS, 1999]). Before the 1990s, daily meteorological weather forecasts for the Polygon region are not available.

28 Anthropologist Eeva Kesküla found similar disposition among Russian-speaking miners working for ArcelorMittal in the Karaganda region (Eeva Kesküla, "Oasis in the Steppe: Health and Masculinity of Kazakhstani Miners," *Central Asian Survey* 37, no. 4 [2018]: 11).

29 Ministry of Justice of the Republic of Kazakhstan, *Labour Code of the Republic of Kazakhstan. Code of the Republic of Kazakhstan Dated 23 November, No. 414-V* [in Russian] (Astana, Kazakhstan: Legal Information System of Regulatory Legal Acts of the Republic of Kazakhstan), https://adilet.zan.kz/eng/docs/K1500000414.

30 Danuta Penkala-Gawęcka, "Shamans, Islam and the State of Medical Policy in Post-Soviet Kazakhstan and Kyrgyzstan," in *The Shamaness in Asia: Gender, Religion and the State*, ed. Davide Torri and Sophie Roche (London: Routledge, 2020), 100–30.

31 The Soviet government sought to eliminate all Kazakh ethno-medical customs that were seen as "backward," dangerous, and in need of transformation, replacing them with a biomedical approach to health (Michaels, *Curative Powers*). Traditional medical beliefs and practices, however, were not eradicated (Danuta Penkala-Gawęcka, "The Way of the Shaman and the Revival of Spiritual Healing in Post-Soviet Kazakhstan and Kyrgyzstan," *Journal of the International Society for Academic Research on Shamanism* 22, no. 1–2 [2014]: 35–59).

32 Alexandr Katsaga, Maksut Kulzhanov, Marina Karanikolos, and Bernd Rechel, *Kazakhstan: Health System Review* (Copenhagen: World Health Organization, on behalf of the European Observatory on Health Systems and Policies, 2012).

33 B. Rechel, M. Ahmedov, B. Akkazieva, A. Katsaga, G. Khodjamurodov, M. McKee, "Lessons from Two Decades of Health Reform in Central Asia," *Health Policy and Planning* 27, no. 4 (2012): 281–7; Bernd Rechel, Erica Richardson, and Martin McKee, eds., *Trends in Health Systems in the Former Soviet Countries* (Copenhagen: World Health Organization on behalf of the European Observatory on Health Systems and Policies, 2014).

34 Katsaga et al., *Kazakhstan: Health System Review*.

35 Francis Amagoh, *Healthcare Policies in Kazakhstan: A Public Sector Reform Perspective* (Singapore: Springer Verlag, 2021).

36 Gulis et al., "Population Health Status of the Republic of Kazakhstan."

37 Katsaga et al., *Kazakhstan: Health System Review*; see also Lazat Spankulova, Marat Karatayev, and Michèle Clarke, "Trends in Socioeconomic Health Inequalities in Kazakhstan: National Household Surveys Analysis," *Communist and Post-Communist Studies* 53, no. 2 (2020): 177–90.

38 Shalkar Adambekov et al., "Health Challenges in Kazakhstan and Central Asia," *Journal of Epidemiology and Community Health* 70 (2016): 104–8. Heart disease and cancer (breast, oesophagus, and lung) are the leading causes of death in the country (Gulis et al., "Population Health Status of the Republic of Kazakhstan"). In comparison with other European countries (Kazakhstan is part of the World Health Organization European Region) mortality from cardiovascular disease is much higher in Kazakhstan than elsewhere in the region, while cancer rates, although lower, increased six percent between 2006 and 2011, especially in industrial regions with

elevated levels of environmental pollutants (Altyn Aringazina, Gabriel Gulis, and John Allegrante, "Public Health Challenges and Priorities for Kazakhstan," *Central Asian Journal of Global Health* 1, no. 1 [2012], https://cajgh.pitt.edu/ojs/index.php/cajgh/article/view/30/47). Life expectancy averages 76.3 years for women and 66.2 years for men (WHO [World Health Organization], *Health Systems in Action: Kazakhstan* [Brussels: World Health Organization European Region/European Observatory on Health Systems and Policies, 2022], https://eurohealthobservatory.who.int/publications/i/health-systems-in-action-kazakhstan-2022).

39 OECD (Organisation for Economic Co-operation and Development), *OECD Reviews of Health Systems: Kazakhstan 2018* (Paris: OECD Publishing, 2018).

40 WHO, *Health Systems in Action*.

41 The historical relationship between experts (scientists or the medical establishment) and local populations on the Polygon mimics the "deflation of expertise," or the increasing global lack of trust between science and society (Vincent Ialenti, *Deep Time Reckoning: How Future Thinking Can Help Earth Now* [Cambridge, MA: MIT Press, 2020], 6). Koianer mistrust and outright rejection of expert knowledge, however, makes sense given the history and people's experiences with authority.

42 Tursynbek's description matched that of a Peace Corps volunteer I met who lived in the regional town where the hospital is. He fractured his ankle and went to the hospital to get treatment, where his initial "prescription" was to soak his foot in half a bucket of vodka. A week later they took an X-ray and reported back that nothing was wrong. He ended up going to Almaty – more than nine hundred miles (fifteen hundred kilometres) south of where he was – to a Western clinic to get help, where the multiple hairline fractures were accurately diagnosed.

43 Nancy Scheper-Hughes, *Death without Weeping: The Violence of Everyday Life in Brazil* (Berkeley: University of California Press, 1992).

44 "Bad faith" can also be understood a form of denial or avoidance, a way to "bury reality" (Don DeLillo, *Americana* [London: Penguin Books, 2006], 334).

45 Masco, "Mutant Ecologies," 517–50.

46 Jake Kosek, "Ecologies of Empire: On the New Uses of the Honeybee," *Cultural Anthropology* 25, no. 4 (2010): 653.

Conclusion

1 Photographer Claudia Heinermann discovered similar findings during interviews with people (Claudia Heinermann, *Siberian Exiles Part III: The Story of Marju and the Legacy of the Atomic Gulag* [Vilnius, Lithuania: KOPA, 2022]).

2 Peter Bradshaw, "After the Apocalypse – Review," *The Guardian*, May 12, 2011, https://www.theguardian.com/film/2011/may/12/after-the-apocalypse-review.

3 Dubrova et al., "Nuclear Weapons Tests and Human Germline Mutation Rate," 1037.
4 Albina Akhmetova, "Geneticheskii Genotsid. Postradavshie ot Semipa-latinskogo Poligona (Kazakhstan) Stat'izgoiami Obshchestva" [Genetic genocide. Victims of the Semipalatinsk test site (Kazakhstan) become social outcasts] *CentrAsia*, August 22, 2003, https://centrasia.org/newsA.php?st=1061504640.
5 Susan Sontag, *Regarding the Pain of Others* (New York: Farrar, Straus and Giroux, 2003).
6 Sontag, *Regarding the Pain of Others*.
7 Peace Corps, "Peace Corps Suspends Program in Kazakhstan," November 18, 2011, https://www.peacecorps.gov/news/library/peace-corps-suspends-program-in-kazakhstan/.
8 Anton Blok, *Radical Innovators: The Blessings of Adversity in Science and Art, 1500-2000* (Cambridge, UK: Polity Press, 2017).
9 Nancy Scheper-Hughes, "A Talent for Life: Reflections on Human Vulnera-bility and Resilience," *Ethnos* 73, no. 1 (2008): 25–56.
10 Marlene Laruelle, ed., *Migration and Social Upheaval as the Face of Globaliza-tion in Central Asia* (Boston, MA: Brill, 2013); Reeves, *Border Work*.
11 See Volodine, *Radiant Terminus*.
12 "About the Channel," 5-Kanal, https://www.5tv.kz/?do=cat&category=about.
13 Hamid Ismailov, *The Dead Lake* (London: Peirene Press Ltd, 2014), 45–6.
14 Mikhail Alexandrov, *Uneasy Alliance: Relations between Russia and Kazakhstan in the Post-Soviet Era, 1992–1997* (Westport, CT: Greenwood Press, 1999).
15 "Uranium and Nuclear Power in Kazakhstan," World Nuclear Association, updated August 2023, https://world-nuclear.org/information-library/country-profiles/countries-g-n/kazakhstan.aspx.
16 IAEA, "IAEA Low Enriched Uranium (LEU) Bank." 2023. https://www.iaea.org/topics/iaea-low-enriched-uranium-bank.
17 UNHRC (United Nations Human Rights Council), *Report of the Special Rapporteur on the Implications for Human Rights of the Environmentally Sound Management and Disposal of Hazardous Substances and Wastes: Mission to Ka-zakhstan* (Geneva: United Nations, 2015).
18 OECD (Organisation for Economic Co-operation and Development), *Kazakh-stan: Review of the Central Administration, OECD Public Governance Reviews* (Paris: OECD Publishing, 2014).
19 UNHRC, *Report of the Special Rapporteur on the Implications for Human Rights of the Environmentally Sound Management and Disposal of Hazardous Sub-stances and Wastes*.
20 Arkady Strugatsky and Boris Strugatsky, *Roadside Picnic* (London: Gollancz, 2007 [1972]).

Bibliography

Abashin, Sergei. *Sovetskii Kishlak: Mezhdu Kolonialismom i Modernizatsiei* [Soviet Kishlak: Between colonialism and modernization]. Moscow: Novoe Literaturnoe Obozrenie, 2015.

Abu-Lughod, Lila. "The Romance of Resistance: Tracing Transformations of Power Through Bedouin Women." *American Ethnologist* 17, no. 1 (1990): 41–55. https://doi.org/10.1525/ae.1990.17.1.02a00030.

Adambekov, Shalkar, Aiym Kaiyrlykyzy, Nurbek Igissinov, and Faina Linkov. "Health Challenges in Kazakhstan and Central Asia." *Journal of Epidemiology and Community Health* 70 (2016): 104–108. https://doi.org/10.1136/jech-2015-206251.

Adushkin, V. Vitaly, and William Leith. *The Containment of Soviet Underground Nuclear Explosions, Open File Report 01-312*. Washington, DC: Department of the Interior Geological Survey, 2001.

Agamben, Giorgio. *Homo Sacer: Sovereign Power and Bare Life*. Stanford, CA: Stanford University Press, 1998.

Agard-Jones, Vanessa. "Bodies in the System." *Small Axe* 17, no. 3 (2013): 182–92. https://doi.org/10.1215/07990537-2378991.

Agency on Statistics of the Republic of Kazakhstan. *Results of the 2009 National Population Census of the Republic of Kazakhstan: Analytical Report*. Astana, Kazakhstan, 2011.

Akhmetova, Albina. "Geneticheskii Genotsid. Postradavshie ot Semipalatinskogo Poligona (Kazakhstan) Stat'izgoiami Obshchestva" [Genetic genocide. Victims of the Semipalatinsk test site (Kazakhstan) become social outcasts]. *CentrAsia* (22 August 2003). https://centrasia.org/newsA.php?st=1061504640.

Alexander, Catherine. "A Chronotope of Expansion: Resisting Spatio-temporal Limits in a Kazakh Nuclear Town." *Ethnos* 88, no. 3 (2020): 467–90. https://www.tandfonline.com/doi/full/10.1080/00141844.2020.1796735.

– "Nettoyer et Tourner la Page: La Renaissance Nucléaire du Kazakhstan" [Cleaning up and moving on: Kazakhstan's nuclear renaissance]. In *Les

Chantiers du Nucléaire, edited by Romain Garcier and Françoise Lafaye, 1–26. Paris: Archives Contemporaines, 2016.

– "Homeless in the Homeland: Housing Protests in Kazakhstan." *Critique of Anthropology* 38, no. 2 (2018): 204–20. https://doi.org/10.1177/0308275x18758872.

– "Value, Relations, and Changing Bodies: Privatization and Property Rights in Kazakhstan." In *Property in Question: Value Transformation in the Global Economy*, edited by Caroline Humphrey and Katherine Verdery, 251–75. New York: Routledge, 2004.

Alexandrov, Mikhail. *Uneasy Alliance: Relations between Russia and Kazakhstan in the Post-Soviet Era, 1992–1997*. Westport, CT: Greenwood Press, 1999.

Alexievich, Svetlana. *Voices from Chernobyl: The Oral History of a Nuclear Disaster*. New York: Picador, 2006.

Alexis-Martin, Becky. *Disarming Doomsday: The Human Impact of Nuclear Weapons Since Hiroshima*. London: Pluto Press, 2019.

Aliyakparov, M., N. Kozachenko, A. Abisheva, R. Dosmagambetova, and I. Galstrev. *Mediko-Ekologicheskie Problemy Karagandinskogo Regiona: Populiatsionnye Issledovaniia Poslednego Desiatiletiia* [Medical and ecological problems of the Karaganda region: Population studies of the last decade]. Karaganda, Kazakhstan: Agenstvo Respubliki Kazakhstan po Delam Zdravookhraneniya, 2001.

Alimaev, Iliya, and Roy Behnke. "Ideology, Land Tenure and Livestock Mobility in Kazakhstan." In *Fragmentation in Semi-Arid and Arid Landscapes*, edited by Kathleen A. Galvin, Robin S. Reid, Roy H. Behnke Jr., and N. Thompson Hobbs, 151–78. London: Springer, 2008.

Amagoh, Francis. *Healthcare Policies in Kazakhstan: A Public Sector Reform Perspective*. Singapore: Springer Verlag, 2021.

Appel, Hilary, and Mitchell Orenstein. "Why did Neoliberalism Triumph and Endure in the Post-Communist World?" *Comparative Politics* 48, no. 3 (2016): 313–31. https://doi.org/10.5129/001041516818254419.

Aringazina, Altyn, Gabriel Gulis, and John Allegrante. "Public Health Challenges and Priorities for Kazakhstan." *Central Asian Journal of Global Health* 1, no. 1 (2012). https://cajgh.pitt.edu/ojs/index.php/cajgh/article/view/30/47.

Arndt, Melanie and Laurent Coumel. "A Green End to the Red Empire? Ecological Mobilizations in the Soviet Union and Its Successor States, 1950–2000: A Decentralized Approach." *Ab Imperio* 1 (2019): 105–24.

Atchabarov, Aidar. "Kainar Syndrome: History of the First Epidemiological Case-Control Study of the Effects of Radiation and Malnutrition." *Central Asian Journal of Global Health* 4, no. 1 (2015): 221. https://doi.org/10.5195/cajgh.2015.221.

Atchabarov, Bakiia. *Zablushdeniia, Lozh' i Istina po Voprosu Otsenki Vliianiia na Zdorov'e Liudei Ispytaniia Atomnogo Oruzhii na Semipalatinskom Iadernom Poligone* [Misconceptions, lies and truths on the issue of assessing the health impact of nuclear weapons testing at the Semipalatinsk nuclear test site]. Almaty, Kazakhstan: Karzhy-Karazhat, 2002.

Auyero, Javier, and Debora Swistun. *Flammable: Environmental Suffering in an Argentine Shantytown*. New York: Oxford University Press, 2009.

Baiburin, Albert. *The Soviet Passport: The History, Nature and Uses of the Internal Passport in the USSR*. Cambridge, UK: Polity Press, 2021.

Balmukhanov, Saim, J.N. Abdrakhmanov, Timur Balmukhanov, Boris Gusev, Natalya Kurakina, and Tolegen Raisov. *Medical Effects and Dosimetric Data from Nuclear Tests at the Semipalatinsk Test Site*. Bethesda, MD: Armed Forces Radiobiology Research Institute, 2006 [1999].

– *The Semipalatinsk Nuclear Test Site: Through My Own Eyes*. Fort Belvoir, VA: Defense Technical Information Center, 2014.

– *Medical Effects and Dosimetric Data from Nuclear Tests at the Semipalatinsk Test Site: Technical Report*. Fort Belvoir, VA: Defense Threat Reduction Agency, 2006.

Balmukhanov, Saim, Galina Raissova, and Timor Balmukhanov. *Three Generations of the Semipalatinsk Affected to the Radiation*. Almaty, Kazakhstan: Sakshy Press, 2002.

Balonov, Mikhail. "Review of Chernobyl: Consequences of the Catastrophe for People and the Environment by Alexey V. Yablokov, Vassily B. Nesterenko, and Alexey V. Nesterenko." *Annals of the New York Academy of Sciences* 1181 (December 2009). http://www.nyas.org/asset.axd?id=8b4c4bfc-3b35-434f-8a5c-ee5579d11dbb&t=634507382459270000.

Barker, Holly. *Bravo for the Marshallese: Regaining Control in a Post-nuclear, Post-colonial World*. Belmont, CA: Wadsworth/Thomson, 2004.

Barnes, Steven. *Death and Redemption: The Gulag and the Shaping of Soviet Society*. Princeton, NJ: Princeton University Press, 2011.

Basso, Keith. *Wisdom Sits in Places: Landscape and Language Among the Western Apache*. Albuquerque: University of New Mexico Press, 1996.

Bauer, Susanne. "Fallout Memory Trajectories at Semipalatinsk: Reassembling the Post-Soviet Past." In *Tracing the Atom: Nuclear Legacies in Russia and Central Asia*, edited by Susanne Bauer and Tanja Penter, 196–216. New York: Routledge, 2022.

– "Beyond the Nuclear Epicenter: Health Research, Knowledge Infrastructures and Secrecy at Semipalatinsk." *Cahiers du Monde Russe* 60, no. 2–3 (2019): 493–516. https://doi.org/10.4000/monderusse.11271.

– "Radiation Science After the Cold War. The Politics of Measurement, Risk and Compensation in Kazakhstan." In *Health, Technologies, and Politics in Post-Soviet Settings: Navigating Uncertainties*, edited by Olga Zvonareva, Evgeniya Popova, and Klasien Horstman, 225–49. Cham, Switzerland: Palgrave Macmillan, 2017.

– "Tracing Mutations: Biodosimetry Tools in Post–Cold War Radiation Epidemiology." In *Making Mutations: Objects, Practices, Contexts*, edited by Luis Campos and Alexander von Schwerin, 209–221. Berlin: Max Planck Institute for the History of Science, 2010.

Bauer, Susanne, Boris I. Gusev, Ludmila M. Pivina, Kazbek N. Apsalikov, and Bernd Grosche. "Radiation Exposure Due to Local Fallout from Soviet Atmospheric Nuclear Weapons Testing in Kazakhstan: Solid Cancer Mortality in the Semipalatinsk Historical Cohort, 1960–1999." *Radiation Research* 164, no. 4 (2005): 409–19. https://doi.org/10.1667/rr3423.1.

Bauman, Zygmunt. *Wasted Lives: Modernity and Its Outcasts*. Cambridge, UK: Polity Press, 2004.

Beck, Ulrich. *The Brave New World of Work*. Cambridge, UK: Polity Press, 2000.

Becker, Charles, Jeffery Hill, and Sultan Muratov. "Brighter than a Million Suns: Contemporary Health Consequences of Atomic Testing in the Semipalatinsk Nuclear Polygon." *IPPA Working Paper Series: Working Paper #70*. Bishkek, Kyrgyzstan: University of Central Asia, 2022.

Benjamin, Walter. "On the Concept of History." In *Walter Benjamin: Selected Writings, Volume 4: 1938–1940*, edited by Howard Eiland and Michael W. Jennings, 392. Cambridge, MA: Harvard University Press, 2003.

Bensaude-Vincent, Bernadette, Soraya Boudia, and Kyoko Sato, eds. *Living in a Nuclear World: From Fukushima to Hiroshima*. New York: Routledge, 2022.

Bergkvist, Nils-Olov, and Ragnhild Ferm. *Nuclear Explosions 1945–1998*. Stockholm: Sipri Stockholm International Peace Research Institute; Defense Research Establishment Division of Systems and Underwater Technology, 2000.

Bernard, Russell. *Research Methods in Anthropology. Qualitative and Quantitative Approaches*. 6th ed. Lanham, MD: Rowman & Littlefield, 2017.

Bertell, Rosalie. "Chernobyl: An Unbelievable Failure to Help." *International Journal of Health Services* 38, no. 3 (2008): 543–60. https://doi.org/10.2190/hs.38.3.i.

Beyer, Judith and Peter Finke. "Practices of Traditionalization in Central Asia." *Central Asian Survey* 38, no. 3 (2019): 310–328. https://doi.org/10.1080/02634937.2019.1636766.

Binder, Otto. "How Nuclear Radiation Can Change Our Race." *Mechanix Illustrated*, December 1953.

Bissenova, Alima. "The Fortress and the Frontier: Mobility, Culture, and Class in Almaty and Astana." *Europe-Asia Studies* 69, no. 4 (2017): 642–67. https://doi.org/10.1080/09668136.2017.1325445.

Blok, Anton. *Radical Innovators: The Blessings of Adversity in Science and Art, 1500–2000*. Cambridge, UK: Polity Press, 2017.

Borofsky, Robert. "Public Anthropology. Where To? What Next?" *Anthropology News* 41, no. 5 (2000): 9–10. https://doi.org/10.1111/an.2000.41.5.9.

Botev, B. M. "Ministerstvo Oborony v Atomnom Proekte" [Ministry of Defense in the Atomic Project]. *Atom* 81 (2019): 6–13.

Boudia, Soraya, and Nathalie Jas, eds. *Powerless Science? Science and Politics in a Toxic World*. New York: Berghahn, 2014.

Bourdieu, Pierre. "The Forms of Capital." In *Handbook of Theory and Research for the Sociology of Education*, edited by John G. Richardson, 241–58. New York: Greenwood Press, 1986.

Boym, Svetlana. *The Future of Nostalgia*. New York: Basic Books, 2001.

Boztayev, Keshim. *Sindrom Kainara* [Kainar syndrome]. Almaty, Kazakhstan: Atamura, 1994.

Bradshaw, Peter. "After the Apocalypse – Review." *The Guardian*. May 12, 2011. https://www.theguardian.com/film/2011/may/12/after-the -apocalypse-review.

Breman, Jan. "A Bogus Concept?" *New Left Review* 84 (2013): 130–8. https:// newleftreview.org/issues/ii84/articles/jan-breman-a-bogus-concept.

– "A Short History of the Informal Economy." *Global Labour Journal* 14, no. 1 (2023): 21–39. https://doi.org/10.15173/glj.v14i1.5277.

Bromet, Evelyn. "Mental Health Consequences of the Chernobyl Disaster." *Journal of Radiological Protection* 32, no. 1 (2012): 71–5. https://doi.org /10.1088/0952-4746/32/1/n71.

Brown, Kate. *A Biography of No Place: From Ethnic Borderland to Soviet Heartland.* Cambridge, MA: Harvard University Press, 2004.

– "Gridded Lives: Why Kazakhstan and Montana are Nearly the Same Place." *The American Historical Review* 106, no. 1 (2001): 17–48. https://doi .org/10.2307/2652223.

– *Manual for Survival: A Chernobyl Guide to the Future.* New York: W.W. Norton, 2019.

– *Plutopia: Nuclear Families, Atomic Cities, and the Great Soviet and American Plutonium Disasters.* Oxford: Oxford University Press, 2013.

Brunn, Stanley. "Fifty Years of Soviet Nuclear Testing in Semipalatinsk, Kazakhstan: Juxtaposed Worlds of Blasts and Silences, Security and Risks, Denials and Memory." In *Engineering Earth: The Impacts of Megaengineering Projects*, edited by Stanley Brunn, 1789–818. Dordrecht, NL: Springer, 2011.

Bruno, Andy. *The Nature of Soviet Power: An Arctic Environmental History.* Cambridge, UK: Cambridge University Press, 2016.

Burawoy, Michael and Katherine Verdery, eds. *Uncertain Transition: Ethnographies of Change in the Postsocialist World.* Lanham, MD: Rowman & Littlefield, 1990.

Butler, Judith. *Frames of War: When Is Life Grievable?* New York: Verso, 2009.

Button, Gregory. *Disaster Culture: Knowledge and Uncertainty in the Wake of Human and Environmental Catastrophe.* Walnut Creek, CA: Left Coast Press, 2010.

Butts, Antony, dir. *After the Apocalypse.* DVD. London: Tigerlily Films, 2010.

Callahan, Alice. "How Red Wine Lost Its Health Halo." *The New York Times*, February 17, 2024. https://www.nytimes.com/2024/02/17/well/eat /red-wine-heart-health.html.

Cameron, Sarah. *The Hungry Steppe: Famine, Violence, and the Making of Soviet Kazakhstan.* Ithaca, NY: Cornell University Press, 2018.

188   Bibliography

Carlsen, Tina, Leif E. Peterson, Brant A. Ulsh, Cynthia A. Werner, Kathleen L. Purvis, and Anna C. Sharber. "Radionuclide Contamination at Kazakhstan's Semipalatinsk Test Site: Implications on Human and Ecological Health." *Human and Ecological Risk Assessment* 7, no. 4 (2001): 943–55. https://doi.org/10.1080/20018091094754.

Chari, Sharad and Katherine Verdery. "Thinking Between the Posts: Postcolonialism, Postsocialism, and Ethnography after the Cold War." *Comparative Studies in Society and History* 51, no. 1 (2009): 6–34. https://doi.org/10.1017/s0010417509000024.

Chelcea, Liviu. "Goodbye, Post-Socialism? Stranger Things Beyond the Global East." *Eurasian Geography and Economics* (2023). https://doi.org/10.1080/15387216.2023.2236126.

Chelcea, Liviu, and Oana Druta. "Zombie Socialism and the Rise of Neoliberalism in Post-Socialist Central and Eastern Europe." *Eurasian Geography and Economics* 57, no. 4–5 (2016): 521–44. https://doi.org/10.1080/15387216.2016.1266273.

Chernobyl Forum. *Chernobyl's Legacy: Health, Environmental and Socio-Economic Impacts and Recommendations to the Governments of Belarus, the Russian Federation and Ukraine.* Vienna: IAEA, 2005.

Chynybaeva, Baktygul. "Kazakhstan Opens Secret KGB Archives Amid Moves Toward Decolonization in Central Asia." *Radio Free Europe Radio Liberty*, November 12, 2023. https://www.rferl.org/a/kazakhstan-opens-kgb-archives-russian-criticism/32681381.html.

Clifford, James and George E. Marcus, eds. *Writing Culture: The Poetics and Politics of Ethnography.* 2nd ed. Berkeley: University of California Press, 2010.

Collier, Stephen. *Post-Soviet Social: Neoliberalism, Social Modernity, Biopolitics.* Princeton, NJ: Princeton University Press, 2011.

Collins, Daniel L., Andrew Baum, and Jerome E. Singer. "Coping with Chronic Stress at Three Mile Island: Psychological and Biochemical Evidence." *Health Psychology* 2, no. 2 (1983): 149–66. https://doi.org/10.1037/0278-6133.2.2.149.

Comaroff, Jean, and John Comaroff. "After Labor." *Critical Historical Studies* 7, no. 1 (2020): 87–112. https://doi.org/10.1086/708007.

Coumel, Laurent, and Marc Elie. "A Belated and Tragic Ecological Revolution: Nature, Disasters, and Green Activists in the Soviet Union and the Post-Soviet States, 1960s–2010." *The Soviet and Post-Soviet Review* 40 (2013): 157–65. https://doi.org/10.1163/18763324-04002005.

Coumel, Laurent, Benjamin Guichard, and Walter Sperling. "Mémoires, Nostalgie et Usages Sociaux du Passé dans la Russie Contemporaine." *Le Mouvement Social* 260 (2017): 3–15. https://doi.org/10.3917/lms.260.0003.

Cram, Shannon. *Unmaking the Bomb: Environmental Cleanup and the Politics of Impossibility.* Oakland, CA: University of California Press, 2023.

Creager, Angela. *Life Atomic: A History of Radioisotopes in Science and Medicine.* Chicago, IL: University of Chicago Press, 2013.

CTBTO (Comprehensive Nuclear-Test-Ban Treaty). *On-Site Inspections: The Ultimate Verification Measure.* Vienna: Preparatory Commission for the CTBTO, 2009.

Davé, Bhavna. *Kazakhstan: Ethnicity, Language and Power.* New York: Routledge, 2007.

Davies, Thom, and Abel Polese. "Informality and Survival in Ukraine's Nuclear Landscape: Living with the Risks of Chernobyl." *Journal of Eurasian Studies* 6, no. 1 (2015): 34–45. https://doi.org/10.1016/j.euras.2014.09.002.

Davis, Mike. *Dead Cities and Other Tales.* New York: The New Press, 2002.

– *Planet of Slums.* London: Verso, 2006.

DeLillo, Don. *Americana.* London: Penguin Books, 2006.

Denning, Michael. "Wageless Life." *New Left Review* 66 (2010): 79–97. https://newleftreview.org/issues/ii66/articles/michael-denning-wageless-life.

DeJong-Lambert, William. *The Cold War Politics of Genetic Research: An Introduction to the Lysenko Affair.* Dordrecht, NL: Springer, 2012.

Deleuze, Gilles, and Félix Guattari. *A Thousand Plateaus: Capitalism and Schizophrenia.* Translated by Brian Massumi. Minneapolis: University of Minnesota Press, 1987.

Dronin, Nikolai, and Edward Bellinger. *Climate Dependence and Food Problems in Russia 1900–1990: The Interaction of Climate and Agricultural Policy and Their Effect on Food Problems.* Budapest: Central European University Press, 2005.

Dubrova, Yuri, Rakhmet I. Bersimbaev, Leila B. Djansugurova, Maira K. Tankimanova, Zaure Zh. Mamyrbaeva, Riitta Mustonen, Carita Lindholm, Maj Hultén, and Sisko Salomaa. "Nuclear Weapons Tests and Human Germline Mutation Rate." *Science* 295, no. 5557 (2002): 1037. https://doi.org/10.1126/science.1068102.

Dubrova, Yuri, Valeri N. Nesterov, Nicolay G. Krouchinsky, Vladislav A. Ostapenko, Rita Neumann, David L. Neil, and Alec J. Jeffreys. "Human Minisatellite Mutation Rate after the Chernobyl Accident." *Nature* 380, no. 6576 (1996): 683–6. https://doi.org/10.1038/380683a0.

Dubuisson, Eva-Marie, and Anna Genina. "Claiming an Ancestral Homeland: Kazakh Pilgrimage and Migration in Inner Asia." *Central Asian Survey* 30, no. 3–4 (2011): 469–85. https://doi.org/10.1080/02634937.2011.607963.

Duster, Troy. *Backdoor to Eugenics.* New York: Routledge, 1990.

Dvorak, Greg. *Coral and Concrete: Remembering Kwajalein Atoll Between Japan, America, and the Marshall Islands.* Honolulu: University of Hawai'i Press, 2018.

Dyussembekova, Zhazira. "Kazakh Street Artist Draws Attention to Social and Environmental Issues." *The Astana Times,* July 11, 2016. https://astanatimes.com/2016/07/kazakh-street-artist-draws-attention-to-social-and-environmental-issues/.

Edgerton, Robert. *Sick Societies: Challenging the Myth of Primitive Harmony.* New York: The Free Press, 1992.

Ellegren, Hans, Gabriella Lindgren, Craig Primmer, and Anders Pape Møller. "Fitness Loss and Germline Mutations in Barn Swallows Breeding in Chernobyl." *Nature* 389 (1997): 593–96. https://doi.org/10.1038/39303.

Elie, Marc, "The Soviet Dust Bowl and the Canadian Erosion Experience in the New Lands of Kazakhstan, 1950s–1960s." *Global Environment* 8, no. 2 (2015): 259–92. https://doi.org/10.3197/ge.2015.080202.

Farmer, Paul. "An Anthropology of Structural Violence." *Current Anthropology* 45, no. 3 (2004): 305–25. https://doi.org/10.1086/382250.

Fassin, Didier. *Humanitarian Reason: A Moral History of the Present.* Berkeley: University of California Press, 2012.

– *When Bodies Remember: Experiences and Politics of AIDS in South Africa.* Berkeley: University of California Press, 2007

Féaux de la Croix, Jeanne, Irina Arzhantseva, Jeanine Dagyeli, Eva-Marie Dubuisson, Heinrich Härke, Beatrice Penati, Akira Ueda, and Amanda Wooden. "Roundtable Studying the Anthropocene in Central Asia: The Challenge of Sources and Scales in Human-Environment Relations." *Central Asian Survey* 41, no. 1 (2021): 180–203. https://doi.org/10.1080/02634937.2021.1960797.

Federici, Silvia. *Caliban and the Witch: Women, the Body and Primitive Accumulation.* Brooklyn, NY: Autonomedia, 2018.

Ferguson, James. *Expectations of Modernity: Myths and Meanings of Urban Life on the Zambian Copperbelt.* Berkeley: University of California Press, 1999.

– *Give a Man a Fish: Reflections on the New Politics of Distribution.* Durham, NC: Duke University Press, 2015.

Ferguson, James, and Tania Murray Li. *Beyond the "Proper Job": Political-Economic Analysis after the Century of Labouring Man* (Working Paper 51). Cape Town: PLAAS, UWC, 2018.

Feshbach, Murray, and Alfred Friendly, Jr. *Ecocide in the USSR: Health and Nature Under Siege.* New York: Basic Books, 1992.

Fetterman, David. *Ethnography: Step-by-Step.* Thousand Oaks, CA: Sage, 2010.

Ferret, Carole. "The Ambiguities of the Kazakhs' Nomadic Heritage." *Nomadic Peoples. Special Issue: Heritage Process among Nomadic Pastoralist Groups in Muslim Contexts* 20, no. 2 (2016): 176–99. https://doi.org/10.3197/np.2016.200202.

– "Mobile Pastoralism a Century Apart: Continuity and Change in South-Eastern Kazakhstan, 1910 and 2012." *Central Asian Survey* 37, no. 4 (2018): 503–25. https://doi.org/10.1080/02634937.2018.1484698.

Fitzpatrick, Sheila. *Everyday Stalinism: Ordinary Life in Extraordinary Times. Soviet Russia in the 1930s.* Oxford: Oxford University Press, 1999.

Fodor, Éva. "Gender and the Experience of Poverty in Eastern Europe and Russia after 1989." *Communist and Post-Communist Studies* 35, no. 4 (2002): 369–82. https://doi.org/10.1016/s0967-067x(02)00026-0.

Folkers, Cindy. "Fukushima Catastrophe at 6: Normalizing Radiation Exposure Demeans Women and Kids ad Risks Their Health." *Counter Punch*, March 6, 2017. http://www.counterpunch.org/2017/03/06 /fukushima-catastrophe-at-6-normalizing-radiation-exposure-demeans -women-and-kids-and-risks-their-health/.

Foreign Broadcast Information Service. *JPRS Report: Environmental Issues*. Springfield, VA: U.S. Department of Commerce National Technical Information Service, 1990.

Fortun, Kim. *Advocacy after Bhopal: Environmentalism, Disaster, New Global Orders*. Chicago, IL: Chicago University Press, 2001.

– "Ethnography in Late Industrialism." *Cultural Anthropology* 27, no. 3 (2012): 446–64. https://doi.org/10.1111/j.1548-1360.2012.01153.x.

Freeman, Linsay A. *Longing for the Bomb: Oak Ridge and Atomic Nostalgia*. Chapel Hill: University of North Carolina Press, 2015.

Funk, Nanette. "Feminist Critiques of Liberalism: Can They Travel East? Their Relevance in Eastern and Central Europe and the Former Soviet Union." *Signs* 29, no. 3 (2004): 695–726. https://doi.org/10.1086/381105.

Furstenberg, Saipira. "Applying a Global Governance Agenda in Post-Soviet States: The Case of EITI in Kazakhstan and Kyrgyzstan." PhD diss., University of Exeter, 2017.

Gal, Susan, and Gail Kligman. *The Politics of Gender after Socialism: A Comparative-Historical Essay*. Princeton, NJ: Princeton University Press, 2000.

Geist, Edward. *Armageddon Insurance: Civil Defense in the United States and Soviet Union, 1945–1991*. Chapel Hill: The University of North Carolina Press, 2019.

Genz, Joseph. *Breaking the Shell: Voyaging from Nuclear Refugees to People of the Sea in the Marshall Islands*. Honolulu: University of Hawai'i Press, 2018.

Ginzburg, Eugenia. *Journey into the Whirlwind*. New York: Harcourt, Brace & World, 1967.

Giroux, Henry. "Reading Hurricane Katrina: Race, Class, and the Biopolitics of Disposability." *College Literature* 33, no. 3 (2006): 171–96. https://doi .org/10.1353/lit.2006.0037.

Goldstein, Donna. "Experimentalité: Pharmaceutical Insights into Anthropology's Epistemologically Fractured Self." In *Medicine and the Politics of Knowledge*, edited by Susan Levine, 119–52. Cape Town: HSRC Press, 2012.

– "Invisible Harm: Science, Subjectivity and the Things We Cannot See." *Culture, Theory and Critique* 54, no. 4 (2017): 321–9. https://doi.org/10.1080 /14735784.2017.1365310.

– *Laughter Out of Place: Race, Class, Violence, and Sexuality in a Rio Shantytown*. 2nd ed. Berkeley: University of California Press, 2013.

– "Toxic Uncertainties of a Nuclear Era: Anthropology, History, Memoir." *American Ethnologist* 41, no. 3 (2014): 579–84. https://doi.org/10.1111/amet.12087.

Goldstein, Donna M., and Kira Hall. "Mass Hysteria in Le Roy, New York: How Brain Experts Materialized Truth and Outscienced Environmental Inquiry." *American Ethnologist* 42, no. 4 (2015): 640–57. https://doi.org /10.1111/amet.12161.

Goldstein, Donna, and Magdalena E. Stawkowski. "James V. Neel and Yuri E. Dubrova: Cold War Debates and the Genetic Effects of Low-Dose Radiation." *Journal of the History of Biology* 48, no. 1 (2015): 67–98. https:// doi.org/10.1007/s10739-014-9385-0.

Gouré, Leon. *The Medical Aspects of the Chernobyl Nuclear Reactor Accident, Draft Report. Prepared for the Defense Nuclear Agency and OSD/Net Assessment.* Leon Gouré Papers, Box 15.7. Hoover Institution Archives. Stanford, CA: Stanford University Press, 1987.

Graeber, David. "Culture as Creative Refusal." *Cambridge Journal of Anthropology* 31, no. 2 (2013): 1–19. https://doi.org/10.3167/ca.2013.310201.

Grant, Bruce. *In the Soviet House of Culture: A Century of Perestroikas.* Princeton, NJ: Princeton University Press, 1995.

Greene, Gayle. "Science with a Skew: The Nuclear Power Industry after Chernobyl and Fukushima." *The Asia-Pacific Journal* 10, no. 1 (2012): 3. https://apjjf.org/-Gayle-Greene/3672/article.pdf.

– *The Woman Who Knew Too Much: Alice Stewart and the Secrets of Radiation.* Ann Arbor: University of Michigan Press, 1999.

Grosche, Bernd. "Semipalatinsk Test Site: Introduction." *Radiation and Environmental Biophysics* 41, no. 1 (2002): 53–5. https://doi.org/10.1007 /s00411-002-0141-z.

Guha, Ranajit. *Elementary Aspects of Peasant Insurgency in Colonial India.* Delhi: Oxford University Press, 1983.

Gulis, Gabriel, Altyn Aringazina, Zhamilya Sangilbayeva, Kalel Zhan, Evelyne de Leeuw, and John, Allegrante. "Population Health Status of the Republic of Kazakhstan: Trends and Implications for Public Health Policy." *International Journal of Environmental Research and Public Health* 18, no. 22 (2021): 12235. https://doi.org/10.3390/ijerph182212235.

Gusev, B., R. Rosenson, and Z. Abylkassimova. "The Semipalatinsk Nuclear Test Site: A First Analysis of Solid Cancer Incidence (Selected Sites) Due to Test-Related Radiation." *Radiation and Environmental Biophysics* 37, no. 3 (1998): 209–14. https://doi.org/10.1007/s004110050119.

Gusev, Boris, Zhibek Abylkassimova, and Kazbek Apsalikov. "The Semipalatinsk Nuclear Test Site: A First Assessment of the Radiological Situation and the Test-Related Radiation Doses in the Surrounding Territories." *Radiation and Environmental Biophysics* 36, no. 3 (1997): 201–4. https://doi.org/10.1007/s004110050072.

Gusterson, Hugh. *Nuclear Rites: A Weapons Laboratory at the End of the Cold War.* Berkeley: University of California Press, 1996.

Guzeeva, Milana. "Nevidimye Miru Dozy" [Doses invisible to the world]. *Vremya*, April 27, 2013. http://www.time.kz/articles/risk/2013/04/27/nevidimie-miru-dozi.

Hacking, Ian. "Making Up People." In *Reconstructing Individualism: Autonomy, Individuality and the Self in Western Thought*, edited by Thomas C. Heller, Morton Sosna, and David E. Wellbery, 222–36. Stanford, CA: Stanford University Press, 1986.

Hamblin, Jacob. *Arming Mother Nature: The Birth of Catastrophic Environmentalism*. New York: Oxford University Press, 2013.

Hamblin, Jacob, and Linda Richards, eds. *Making the Unseen Visible: Science and the Contested Histories of Radiation Exposure*. Corvallis, OR: Oregon State University, 2023.

Hann, Chris, and Jonathan Parry, eds. *Industrial Labor on the Margins of Capitalism: Precarity, Class, and the Neoliberal Subject*. New York: Berghahn, 2018.

Hanson, Margaret. "Legalized Rent-Seeking: Eminent Domain in Kazakhstan." *Cornell International Law Journal* 50, no. 1 (2017): 15–46. https://doi.org/10.31228/osf.io/2czfb.

Haraway, Donna. *When Species Meet*. Minneapolis: University of Minnesota Pres, 2008.

Harrell, Eben, and David E. Hoffman. *Plutonium Mountain: Inside the 17-Year Mission to Secure a Dangerous Legacy of Soviet Nuclear Testing*. Cambridge, MA: The Project on Managing the Atom, Belfer Center for Science and International Affairs, Harvard University, 2013.

Hart, Keith. "The Informal Economy." *The Cambridge Journal of Anthropology* 10, no. 2 (1985): 54–8. https://www.jstor.org/stable/23816368.

– "Informal Income Opportunities and Urban Employment in Ghana." *The Journal of Modern African Studies* 11, no. 1 (1973): 61–89. https://doi.org/10.1017/s0022278x00008089.

Harvey, David. *The Condition of Postmodernity*. Cambridge, UK: Blackwell, 1990.

– "Neoliberalism as Creative Destruction." *The Annals of the American Academy of Political and Social Science* 610 (2007): 22–44. https://doi.org/10.1177/0002716206296780.

Hauck, Markus, Gulzhan Artykbaeva, Tamara Zozulya, and Choimaa Dalamsuren. "Pastoral Livestock Husbandry and Rural Livelihoods in the Forest-Steppe of East Kazakhstan." *Journal of Arid Environments* 133 (2016): 102–11. https://doi.org/10.1016/j.jaridenv.2016.05.009.

Hayward, Daniel. "Kazakhstan-Context and Land Governance." *Land Portal*, 2022. https://landportal.org/book/narratives/2022/kazakhstan#ref16.

Hecht, Gabrielle. *Being Nuclear: Africans and the Global Uranium Trade*. Cambridge, MA: MIT Press, 2012.

– "Nuclear Ontologies." *Constellations* 13, no. 3 (2006): 320–31. https://doi.org/10.1111/j.1467-8675.2006.00404.x.

Heinermann, Claudia. *Siberian Exiles Part III: The Story of Marju and the Legacy of the Atomic Gulag*. Vilnius, Lithuania: KOPA, 2022.

Henig, David, and Nicolette Makovicky, eds. *Economies of Labour after Socialism*. Oxford: Oxford University Press, 2013.

Hennaoui, Leila, and Marzhan Nurzhan. "Dealing with a Nuclear Past: Revisiting the Cases of Algeria and Kazakhstan through a Decolonial Lens." *The International Spectator* 58, no. 4 (2023): 91–109. https://doi.org/10.1080/03932729.2023.2234817.

Hill, Christopher Robert. "Britain, West Africa and 'the New Nuclear Imperialism': Decolonisation and Development during French Tests." *Contemporary British History* 33, no. 2 (2019): 274–89. https://doi.org/10.1080/13619462.2018.1519426.

Holloway, David. *Stalin and the Bomb: The Soviet Union and Atomic Energy, 1939–1956*. New Haven, CT: Yale University Press, 1994.

Högselius, Per, and Achim Klüpperlberg. *The Soviet Nuclear Archipelago: A Historical Geography of Atomic-Powered Communism*. Budapest: Central European University Press, 2024.

Humphrey, Caroline. *The Unmaking of the Soviet Life: Everyday Economies after Socialism*. Ithaca, NY: Cornell University Press, 2002.

Humphrey, Carolina and David Sneath. *The End of Nomadism? Society, State and the Environment in Inner Asia*. Durham, NC: Duke University Press, 1999.

IAEA (International Atomic Energy Agency). *IAEA Low Enriched Uranium (LEU) Bank*. 2023. https://www.iaea.org/topics/iaea-low-enriched-uranium-bank.

– *One Decade after Chernobyl: Summing Up the Consequences of the Accident: Proceedings of an International Conference on One Decade After Chernobyl: Summing Up the Consequences of the Accident*. Vienna: IAEA, 1996.

– *Radiological Conditions at the Semipalatinsk Test Site, Kazakhstan: Preliminary Assessment and Recommendations for Further Study. Radiological Assessment Reports Series 3*. Vienna: IAEA, 1998.

Ialenti, Vincent. *Deep Time Reckoning: How Future Thinking Can Help Earth Now*. Cambridge, MA: MIT Press, 2020.

ILO (International Labour Organization). *World Employment and Social Outlook: Trends 2022*. Geneva: International Labour Office, 2022.

– *World Employment and Social Outlook: Trends 2018*. Geneva: International Labour Office, 2018.

Il'in, L.A., and O.A. Pavlovskii. "Radiological Consequences of the Chernobyl Accident and the Measures Implemented to Mitigate Them." *Soviet Atomic Energy* 65, no. 2 (August 1988): 667–77. https://doi.org/10.1007/bf01270809.

Institute of Biophysics of the USSR Academy of Medical Sciences. "Vypiska iz Otchota Resul'taty Naucheneniya Naucheneniia Vozdeistviia Radioaktivnykh Osadkov na Ob'ekty Vneshnei Sredy i Sostaiane Zdrovia Naseleniia Itogi " [The results of studying the impact of radioactive fallout on environmental objects and the health of the population] *Archive in Semey Scientific Research Institute for Radiation Medicine and Ecology*, 1958.

Ismailbekova, Aksana. "Migration and Patrilineal Descent: The Role of Women in Kyrgyzstan." *Central Asian Survey* 33, no. 3 (2014): 375–89. https://doi.org/10.1080/02634937.2014.961305.

Ismailov, Hamid. *The Dead Lake*. London: Peirene Press Ltd., 2014.

Jacobs, Robert. *Nuclear Bodies: The Global Hibakusha*. New Haven, CT: Yale University Press, 2022.

Jain, S. Lochlann. *Malignant: How Cancer Becomes Us*. Berkeley: University of California Press, 2013.

Jaworowski, Zbigniew. "Observations on Chernobyl After 25 Years of Radiophobia." *21st Century Science & Technology* (Summer 2010): 30–45. https://21sci-tech.com/Articles_2010/Summer_2010/Observations _Chernobyl.pdf.

Johnston, Barbara Rose, and Holly Barker. *Consequential Damages of Nuclear War: The Rongelap Report*. Walnut Creek, CA: Left Coast Press, 2008.

Johnston, Barbara Rose, ed. *Half-Lives and Half-Truths: Confronting the Radioactive Legacies of the Cold War*. Santa Fe, NM: School for Advanced Research Press, 2007.

Jones-Luong, Pauline, and Erika Weinthal. *Oil is Not a Curse: Ownership Structure and Institutions in Soviet Successor States*. New York: Cambridge University Press, 2010.

Josephson, Paul. "Industrial Deserts: Industry, Science and the Destruction of Nature in the Soviet Union." *Slavonic and East European Review* 85, no. 2 (April 2007). https://doi.org/10.1353/see.2007.0073.

Josephson, Paul, Nicolai Dronin, Ruben Mnatsakanian, Aleh Cherp, Dmitry Efremenko, and Vladislav Larin, eds. *An Environmental History of Russia*. Cambridge, UK: Cambridge University Press, 2013.

Jumazhanova, Gulzhanar, Gulnar Tursungozhinova, Oxana Belenko, Marzhan Iskakova, and Aray Amanova. "Ecological Consciousness of a Personality Living in an Ecologically Unfavorable Region." *International Journal of Environmental and Science Education* 11, no. 7 (2016): 1469–78. http://www .ijese.net/makale_indir/IJESE_223_article_57398db5b676a.pdf.

Junisbai, Barbara. "A Tale of Two Kazakhstans: Sources of Political Cleavage and Conflict in the Post-Soviet Period." *Europe-Asia Studies* 62, no. 2 (2010): 235–69. https://doi.org/10.1080/09668130903506813.

Kadyrzhanov, K., and Lukashenko, S. "Radioactivity in Kazakhstan. Cases and Consequences." In *Environmental Protection Against Radioactive Pollution*, edited by Nevzat Birsen and Kairat Kadyrzhanov, 11–18. Dordrecht, NL: Kluwer Academic Publishers, 2003.

Kandiyoti, Deniz. "The Politics of Gender and the Soviet Paradox: Neither Colonized, Nor Modern?" *Central Asian Survey* 26, no. 4 (2008): 601–23. https://doi.org/10.1080/02634930802018521.

Kassenova, Togzhan. *Atomic Steppe: How Kazakhstan Gave Up the Bomb.* Stanford, CA: Stanford University Press, 2022.

Kassymbekova, Botakoz, and Aminat Chokobaeva. "On Writing Soviet History of Central Asia: Frameworks, Challenges, Prospects." *Central Asian Survey* 40, no. 4 (2021): 483–503. https://doi.org/10.1080/02634937.2021.1976728.

Katayama, Hiroaki, Kazbek N. Apsalikov, Boris I. Gusev, Boris Galich, Madina Madieva, Gulsum Koshpessova, Asel Abdikarimova, and Masaharu Hoshi. "An Attempt to Develop a Database for Epidemiological Research in Semipalatinsk." *Journal of Radiation Research* 47, no. 1 (2006): A189–A197. https://doi.org/10.1269/jrr.47.a189.

Katsaga, Alexandr, Maksut Kulzhanov, Marina Karanikolos, and Bernd Rechel. "Kazakhstan: Health System Review." *Copenhagen: World Health Organization, on behalf of the European Observatory on Health Systems and Policies*, 2012.

Kawano, Noriyuki, Kyoko Hirabayashi, Masatsugu Matsuo, Yasuyuki Taooka, Takashi Hiraoka, Kazbek N. Apsalikov, Talgat Moldagaliev, and Masaharu Hoshi. "Human Suffering Effects of Nuclear Tests at Semipalatinsk, Kazakhstan: Established On the Basis of Questionnaire Surveys." *Journal of Radiation Research* 47, Supplement A (2006): A209–217. https://doi.org/10.1269/jrr.47.a209.

Kayser, Lis. "Nuclear Nostalgia: Remembering the Nuclear Age on the Hao Atoll, French Polynesia." PhD diss., University of Aarhus, 2023.

Kesküla, Eeva. "Oasis in the Steppe: Health and Masculinity of Kazakhstani Miners." *Central Asian Survey* 37, no. 4 (2018): 546–62.

Khalid, Adeeb. "Backwardness and the Quest for Civilization: Early Soviet Central Asia in Comparative Perspective." *Slavic Review* 65, no. 2 (2006): 231–51. https://doi.org/10.2307/4148591.

– *Central Asia: A New History from the Imperial Conquests to the Present.* Princeton, NJ: Princeton University Press, 2021.

Kirchhof, Astrid Mignon, and J.R. McNeill. *Nature and the Iron Curtain: Environmental Policy and Social Movements in Communist and Capitalist Countries 1945–1990.* Pittsburgh, PA: Pittsburgh University Press, 2019.

Kligman, Gail. *The Politics of Duplicity: Controlling Reproduction in Ceausescu's Romania.* Berkeley: University of California Press, 1998.

Koch, Natalie. "Bordering on the Modern: Power, Practice and Exclusion in Astana." *Transactions* 39, no. 3 (2013): 432–43. https://doi.org/10.1111/tran.12031.

– *The Geopolitics of Spectacle: Space, Synecdoche, and the New Capitals of Asia.* Ithaca, NY: Cornell University Press, 2018.

Koch, Natalie, and Kristopher White. "Cowboys, Gangsters, and Rural Bumpkins: Constructing the 'Other' in Kazakhstan's 'Texas.'" In *Legitimacy, Symbols, and Social Changes*, edited by M. Laruelle, 181–207. Lanham, MD: Lexington Books, 2016.

Kopack, Robert. "Rocket Wastelands in Kazakhstan: Scientific Authoritarianism and the Baikonur Cosmodrome." *Annals of the American Association of Geographers* 109, no. 2 (2019): 556–67. https://doi.org/10.1080/24694452.2018.1507817.

Korostelyova, Yuna. "Regional Pathology: How Long-Term Nuclear Weapons Tests Have Affected the Health of People Living Nearby." [In Russian.] Polygon. n.d. https://polygon.vlast.kz/health.

Kosek, Jake. "Ecologies of Empire: On the New Uses of the Honeybee." *Cultural Anthropology* 25, no. 4 (2010): 650–78. https://doi.org/10.1111/j.1548-1360.2010.01073.x.

Kotkin, Stephen. *Magnetic Mountain: Stalinism as a Civilization.* Berkeley: University of California Press.

Kret, Abigail. " 'We Unite with Knowledge': The Peoples' Friendship University and Soviet Education for the Third World." *Comparative Studies of South Asia, Africa, and the Middle East* 33, no. 2 (2013): 239–56. https://doi.org/10.1215/1089201x-2322516.

Kuchinskaya, Olga. *The Politics of Invisibility: Public Knowledge about Radiation Health Effects after Chernobyl.* Cambridge, MA: MIT Press, 2014.

Kudaibergenova, Diana. "Between the State and the Artist: Representations of Femininity and Masculinity in the Formation of Ideas of the Nation in Central Asia." *Nationalities Papers* 44, no. 2 (2018): 225–46. https://doi.org/10.1080/00905992.2015.1057559.

– "Project Kelin: Marriage, Women, and Re-Traditionalization in Post-Soviet Kazakhstan." In *Women of Asia: Globalization, Development, and Gender Equity,* edited by Mehrangiz Najafizadeh and Linda Lindsey, 379–90. New York: Routledge, 2018.

Kuehnast, Kathleen, and Carol Nechemias, eds. *Post-Soviet Women Encountering Transition: Nation Building, Economic Survival, and Civic Activism.* Baltimore, MD: Johns Hopkins University Press, 2004.

Kuletz, Valerie. *The Tainted Desert: Environmental Ruin in the American West.* New York: Routledge, 1998.

Kundera, Milan. *The Unbearable Lightness of Being.* Trans. Michael Henry Heim. New York: Harper and Row Publishers, 1984.

Kuzgibekova, Almagul, Gulmira Muldayeva, Bibigul Abeuova, Galina Yeryomicheva, Dinagul Baesheva, Venara Tashkenbayeva, Aigul Takirova, Bibigul Tukbekova, Meiram Askarov, and Kamshat Zhumakanova. "The State of Health of Children Living in Adverse Environmental Conditions." *Australasian Medical Journal* 9, no. 12 (2016): 474–80. https://doi.org/10.21767/amj.2016.2682.

Kvartiuk, Vasyl, and Martin Petrick. 2021. "Liberal Land Reform in Kazakhstan? The Effect on Land Rental and Credit Markets." *World Development* 138 (2021): 105285.

Lancet. "Radiophobia." *The Lancet*. November 16, 1935.

Laszczkowski, Mateusz. *City of the Future: Building Space, Modernity, and Urban Change in Astana*. New York: Berghahn, 2016.

Laruelle, Marlene, ed. *Migration and Social Upheaval as the Face of Globalization in Central Asia*. Boston, MA: Brill, 2013.

Lazar, Sian, and Andrew Sanchez. "Understanding Labor Politics in an Age of Precarity." *Dialectical Anthropology* 43, no. 1 (2019): 3–14. https://doi.org/10.1007/s10624-019-09544-7.

Ledeneva, Alena. *How Russia Really Works: The Informal Practices that Shaped Post-Soviet Politics and Business*. Ithaca, NY: Cornell University Press, 2006.

– *Russia's Economy of Favors: Blat, Networking and Informal Exchange*. London: Cambridge University Press, 1998.

Li, Tania Murray. *Land's End: Capitalist Relations on an Indigenous Frontier*. Durham, NC: Duke University Press, 2014.

Lifton, Robert. *Death in Life: Survivors of Hiroshima*. 2nd ed. Chapel Hill: University of North Carolina Press, 1991.

Litvin, Alter and John Keep. *Stalinism: Russian and Western Views at the Turn of the Millennium*. London: Routledge, 2005.

Liu, Morgan. *Under Solomon's Throne: Uzbek Visions of Renewal in Osh*. Pittsburgh, PA: University of Pittsburgh Press, 2012.

Logachev, Vadim. *Iadernye Ispytaniia SSSR. Semipalatinskii Poligon. Fakty, Svidetel'stva, Vospominaniia. Obespechenie Obsshchei i Radiatsionnoi Bezopasnosti Iadernykh Ispytanii* [Nuclear tests of the USSR. Semipalatinsk test site: Facts, evidence, memories. Ensuring general and radiation safety of nuclear tests]. Moscow: IGEM RAN, 1997. http://elib.biblioatom.ru/text/semipalatinskiy-poligon_1997/go,2/.

Logachev, Vadim, L. A. Mikhalikhina, Natalya Darenskaya, A. Matuschchenko, Yuri Stepanov, and O. Shamov. *Population Health in Regions Adjacent to the Semipalatinsk Nuclear Test Site. AFRRI Contract Report 98-94*. Bethesda, MD: Armed Forces Radiobiology Research Institute, 1998.

Logachev, Vadim, and L.A. Mikhalikhina. *Animal Effects from Soviet Atmospheric Nuclear Tests*. Fort Belvoir, VA: Defense Threat Reduction Agency.

Mamonova, Tatyana. *Women's Glasnost vs. Naglost: Stopping Russian Backlash*. Westport, CT: Bergin and Garvey, 1994.

Masco, Joseph. "Mutant Ecologies: Radioactive Life in Post–Cold War New Mexico." *Cultural Anthropology* 19, no. 4 (2004): 517–50. https://doi.org/10.1525/can.2004.19.4.517.

– *The Nuclear Borderlands: The Manhattan Project in Post–Cold War New Mexico*. Princeton, NJ: Princeton University Press, 2006.

Marcus, George. "Ethnography in/of the World System: The Emergence of Multi-Sited Ethnography." *Annual Review of Anthropology* 24 (1995): 95–117. https://doi.org/10.1146/annurev.anthro.24.1.95.

Markabaeva, Akbaya, Susanne Bauer, Ludmila Pivina, Geir Bjorklund, Salvatore Chirumbolo, Aiman Kerimkulova, Yuliya Semenova, and Tatyana Belikhina. "Increased Prevalence of Essential Hypertension in Areas Previously Exposed to Fallout Due to Nuclear Weapons Testing at the Semipalatinsk Test Site, Kazakhstan." *Environmental Research* 167 (2018): 129–35. https://doi.org/10.1016/j.envres.2018.07.016.

Martin, Virginia. *Law and Custom in the Steppe: The Kazakhs of the Middle Horde and Russian Colonialism in the Nineteenth Century.* Richmond, VA: Curzon Press, 2001.

Mazhitova, Zhanna, Aigul Zhalmurzina, Sveta Koganatova, Aitzhan Orazbakov, and Tastanbek Satbai. "Environmental Consequences of Khrushchev's Virgin Land Campaign in Kazakhstan (1950s–1960s)." *E3S Web of Conferences* 285, no. 05036 (2021): 1–12. https://www.e3s-conferences.org/articles/e3sconf/abs/2021/34/e3sconf_uesf2021_05036/e3sconf_uesf2021_05036.html.

McCauley, Martin. *Khrushchev and the Development of Soviet Agriculture: The Virgin Land Programme, 1953–1954.* New York: Holmes and Meier, 1976.

McGranahan, Carole. "Theorizing Refusal: An Introduction." *Cultural Anthropology* 31, no. 3 (2016): 319–25. https://doi.org/10.14506/ca31.3.01.

McMann, Kelly. "The Shrinking of the Welfare state: Central Asians' Assessments of Soviet and Post-Soviet Governance." In *Everyday Life in Central Asia: Past and Present,* edited by Jeff Sahadeo and Russell Zanca, 233–47. Bloomington, IN: Indiana University Press, 2007.

MDG (Millennium Development Goals). *Millennium Development Goals in Kazakhstan.* New York: United Nations Development Program, 2010.

Mendybaeva, Dana. "Zhiteli Karagandinskoi Oblasti Bezhali iz Rabstva" [residents of Karaganda region escaped from slavery]. *Novyi Vestnik,* March 1, 2014. http://nv.kz/2014/03/01/67620/.

Metzl, Jonathan, and Anna Kirkland, eds. *Against Health: How Health Became the New Morality.* New York: New York University Press, 2010.

Michaels, Paula. *Curative Powers: Medicine and Empire in Stalin's Central Asia.* Pittsburgh, PA: University of Pittsburgh Press, 2003.

Mikhailov, V.N., ed. *USSR Nuclear Weapons Tests and Peaceful Nuclear Explosions, 1949 through 1990.* Moscow: Ministry of Atomic Energy and Ministry of Defense of the Russian Federation, 1996.

–, ed. *Iadernye Ispytaniia SSSR. Tom 2: Tekhnologii Iadernykh Ispytanii SSSR. Vozdeistvie na Okruzhaiushchuiu Sredu. Mery po Obespecheniiu Bezopasnosti. Iadernye Poligony i Ploshchadki* [Nuclear tests of the USSR. Volume 2: Nuclear technologies of USSR tests. Environmental impact. Security measures. Nuclear testing sites and platforms] [Sarov, Russia: RFYATS, 1999.

–, ed. *Catalog of Worldwide Nuclear Testing.* New York: Ministry of Atomic Energy of the Russian Federation, Begell-Atom, 1999.

Millar, Kathleen. *Reclaiming the Discarded: Life and Labor on Rio's Garbage Dump.* Durham, NC: Duke University Press, 2018.

Ministry of Justice of the Republic of Kazakhstan. *Labour Code of the Republic of Kazakhstan. Code of the Republic of Kazakhstan Dated 23 November, No. 414-V* [In Russian.] Legal Information System of Regulatory Legal Acts of the Republic of Kazakhstan, 2015. https://adilet.zan.kz/eng/docs/K1500000414.
– *Land Code of the Republic of Kazakhstan. Code of the Republic of Kazakhstan Dated 20 June, 2003, No. 442* [In Russian.] Legal Information System of Regulatory Legal Acts of the Republic of Kazakhstan, 2003. https://adilet .zan.kz/eng/docs/K030000442_.
– *On the Semipalatinsk Nuclear Safety Zone. The Law of the Republic of Kazakhstan Dated July 5, 2023, No. 16-VIII* [In Russian.] Legal Information System of Regulatory Legal Acts of the Republic of Kazakhstan, 2023. https://adilet .zan.kz/eng/docs/Z2300000016.
Mishtal, Joanna. *The Politics of Morality: The Church, the State, and Reproductive Rights in Postsocialist Poland*. Athens, OH: Ohio University Press, 2015.
Moen, Phyllis. *Women's Two Roles: A Contemporary Dilemma*. Westport, CT: Auburn House, 1992.
Monnet, Livia, ed. *Toxic Immanence: Decolonizing Nuclear Legacies and Futures*. Montreal: McGill-Queen's University Press, 2022.
Møller, Anders, J. Erritzøe, F. Karadas, and Timothy Mousseau. "Historical Mutation Rates Predict Susceptibility to Radiation in Chernobyl Birds." *Journal of Evolutionary Biology* 23, no. 10 (2010): 2132–42. https://doi .org/10.1111/j.1420-9101.2010.02074.x.
Møller, Anders, and Timothy Mousseau. "The Effects of Low-Dose Radiation: Soviet Science, the Nuclear Industry – and Independence?" *Significance* 10, no. 1 (2013): 14–19. https://doi.org/10.1111/j.1740-9713.2013.00630.x.
– "Strong Effects of Ionizing Radiation from Chernobyl on Mutation Rates." *Scientific Reports* 5 (2015): 8363. https://doi.org/10.1038/srep0863.
Morgan, William, and William Bair. "Issues in Low Dose Radiation Biology: The Controversy Continues. A Perspective." *Radiation Research* 179, no. 5 (2013): 501–10. https://doi.org/10.1667/rr3306.1.
Morimoto, Ryo. *Nuclear Ghost: Atomic Livelihoods in Fukushima's Gray Zone*. Oakland: University of California Press, 2023.
Morris, Jeremy, and Abel Polese, eds. *The Informal Post-Socialist Economy: Embedded Practices and Livelihoods*. London: Routledge, 2013.
Mousseau, Timothy, and Sarah Todd. "Biological Consequences of Exposure to Radioactive Hydrogen (Tritium): A Comprehensive Survey of the Literature." *SSRN*, 2023. https://papers.ssrn.com/sol3/papers.cfm?abstract_id=4416674.
Mousseau, Timothy, and Anders Møller. Genetic and Ecological Studies of Animals in Chernobyl and Fukushima." *Journal of Heredity* 105, no. 5 (2014): 704–9. https://doi.org/10.1093/jhered/esu040.
Munck, Ronaldo. "The Precariat: A View from the South." *Third World Quarterly* 34, no. 5 (2013): 747–62. https://doi.org/10.1080/01436597.2013.800751.

Murphy, Michelle. *Sick Building Syndrome and the Problem of Uncertainty: Environmental Politics, Technoscience, and Women Workers*. Durham, NC: Duke University Press, 2006.

Nakamura, Nori. "Genetic Effects of Radiation in Atomic-Bomb Survivors and Their Children: Past, Present and Future." *Journal of Radiation Research* 47, supplement B (2006): B67–B73. https://doi.org/10.1269/jrr.47.b67.

Nash, Linda. *Inescapable Ecologies: A History of Environment, Disease, and Knowledge*. Berkeley: University of California Press, 2006.

Nazapary, Joma. *Post-Soviet Chaos: Violence and Dispossession in Kazakhstan*. London: Pluto Press, 2002.

Neel, James. "Two Recent Radiation-Related Genetic False Alarms: Leukemia in West Cumbria, England, and Minisatellite Mutations in Belarus." *Teratology* 59, no. 4 (1999): 302–6. https://doi.org/10.1002/(sici)1096-9926(199904)59:4<302::aid-tera17>3.3.co;2-x.

Nixon, Rob. *Slow Violence and the Environmentalism of the Poor*. Cambridge, MA: Harvard University Press, 2011.

NNC (National Nuclear Center of the Republic of Kazakhstan, Institute of Radiation Safety and Ecology). *Semipalatinskii Ispytatel'nyi Poligon. Sovremennoe Sostoianie* [Semipalatinsk test site. Current state]. Pavlodar, Kazakhstan: Press House, 2017.

– *Semipalatinsk Nuclear Test Site: Present State*. Pavlodar, Kazakhstan: Press House, 2011.

Northrop, Douglas. *Veiled Empire: Gender and Power in Stalinist Central Asia*. Ithaca, NY: Cornell University Press, 2004.

NRC (National Research Council). *Health Risks from Exposure to Low Levels of Ionizing Radiation: BEIR VII, Phase 2*. Washington, DC: National Academies Press, 2006.

OECD (Organisation for Economic Co-operation and Development). *Kazakhstan: Review of the Central Administration, OECD Public Governance Reviews*. Paris: OECD Publishing, 2014.

– *Multi-dimensional Review of Kazakhstan. Volume 1. Initial Assessment*. Paris: OECD Publishing, 2016.

– *Multi-dimensional Review of Kazakhstan: Volume 2. In-Depth Analysis and Recommendations*. Paris: OECD Publishing, 2017.

– *OECD Review of Agricultural Policies: Kazakhstan 2013*. Paris: OECD Publishing, 2013.

– *OECD Reviews of Health Systems: Kazakhstan 2018*. Paris: OECD Publishing, 2018.

Ogawa, Akihiro. *Antinuclear Citizens: Sustainability Policy and Grassroots Activism in Post-Fukushima Japan*. Stanford, CA: Stanford University Press, 2023.

Ohayon, Isabelle. "The Kazakh Famine: The Beginnings of Sedentarization." *Science-Po: On-Line Encyclopedia of Mass Violence*, 2013. https://www

.sciencespo.fr/mass-violence-war-massacre-resistance/en/document
/kazakh-famine-beginnings-sedentarization.html.

– *La Sédentarisation des Kazakhs dans l'URSS de Staline: Collectivisation et Changement Social (1928–1945).* Paris: Maisonneuve et Larose-Institut Français d'études sur l'Asie Centrale, 2006.

Olcott, Martha. *The Kazakhs.* Stanford, CA: Stanford University Press, 1995.

Onaga, Lisa. "Measuring the Particular: The Meanings of Low-Dose Radiation Experiments in Post-1954 Japan." *Positions Asia Critique* 26, no. 2 (2018): 265–304. https://doi.org/10.1215/10679847-4351566.

Ong, Aihwa. *Spirits of Resistance and Capitalist Discipline: Factory Women in Malaysia.* Albany: State University of New York Press, 1987.

Ortner, Sherry. "On Neoliberalism." *Anthropology of This Century*, 2011. http://aotcpress.com/articles/neoliberalism/.

– "Resistance and the Problem of Ethnographic Refusal." *Comparative Studies in Society and History* 37, no. 1 (1995): 173–93. https://doi.org/10.1017/s0010417500019587.

– "Subjectivity and Cultural Critique." *Anthropological Theory* 5, no. 1 (2005): 31–52. https://doi.org/10.1177/1463499605050867.

Ortmeyer, Pat, and Arjun Makhajani. "Worse than We Knew." *The Bulletin of the Atomic Scientists*, November/December 1997, pp. 46–50.

Oushakine, Serguei. *The Patriotism of Despair: Nation, War, and Loss in Russia.* Ithaca, NY: Cornell University Press, 2009.

– "'We're Nostalgic but We're Not Crazy': Retrofitting the Past in Russia." *The Russian Review* 66, no. 3 (2007): 451–82. https://doi.org/10.1111/j.1467-9434.2007.00453.x.

Panicciari, Giulia. "Almaty as a New Kazakh City: Kazakhisation of Urban Spaces after Independence." In *Changing Urban Landscapes: Eastern European and Post-Soviet Cities since 1989*, edited by Marco Buttino, 123–51. Rome: Viella, 2012.

Paxson, Heather. *The Life of Cheese: Crafting Food and Value in America.* Berkeley: University of California Press, 2012.

Peace Corps. "Peace Corps Suspends Program in Kazakhstan." *Peace Corps*, 2011. https://www.peacecorps.gov/news/library/peace-corps-suspends-program-in-kazakhstan/.

Pearce, Fred. "Exposed: Soviet Cover-Up of Nuclear Fallout Worse than Chernobyl." *New Scientist*, March 20, 2017. https://www.newscientist.com/article/2125202-exposed-soviet-cover-up-of-nuclear-fallout-worse-than-chernobyl/.

Pelkmans, Mathijs. *Fragile Conviction: Changing Ideological Landscapes in Urban Kyrgyzstan.* Ithaca, NY: Cornell University Press, 2017.

Penkala-Gawęcka, Danuta. "Shamans, Islam and the State of Medical Policy in Post-Soviet Kazakhstan and Kyrgyzstan." In *The Shamaness in Asia: Gender, Religion and the State*, edited by Davide Torri and Sophie Roche, 100–30. London: Routledge, 2020.

– "The Way of the Shaman and the Revival of Spiritual Healing in Post-Soviet Kazakhstan and Kyrgyzstan." *Journal of the International Society for Academic Research on Shamanism* 22, no. 1–2 (2014): 35–59. https://repozytorium.amu .edu.pl/items/5bb59d6a-1ba5-47a7-b0ed-d4a634d986f8.

Perez Foster, R., Branovan, D., Ukrainsky, G. *Surviving Chernobyl in America: Medical and Mental Health Consequences of the Chernobyl Nuclear Accident.* New York: Media Luna Ltd, 2003.

Perrow, Charles. "Nuclear Denial: From Hiroshima to Fukushima." *Bulletin of the Atomic Scientists* 69, no. 5 (2013): 56–67. https://doi.org/10.1177 /0096340213501369.

Petryna, Adriana. *Life Exposed: Biological Citizens after Chernobyl.* Princeton, NJ: Princeton University Press, 2013.

– *When Experiments Travel: Clinical Trials and the Global Search for Human Subjects.* Princeton, NJ: Princeton University Press, 2009.

Petrick, Martin, and Richard Pomfret. *Agricultural Policies in Kazakhstan. No. 155, IAMO Discussion Papers.* Leibniz Institute of Agricultural Development in Transition Economies, 2016.

Phillips, Sarah. "Half-Lives and Healthy Bodies: Discourses on "Contaminated" Food and Healing in Post-Chernobyl Ukraine." *Food & Foodways* 10 (2002): 27–53. https://doi.org/10.1080/07409710212483.

Pianciola, Niccolo. "Famine in the Steppe: The Collectivization of Agriculture and the Kazakh Herdsmen, 1928–1944." *Cahiers du Monde Russe* 45, no. 1/2 (2004): 137–91. https://doi.org/10.4000/monderusse.2623.

Pitkanen, Laura, and Matthew Farish. "Nuclear Landscapes." *Progress in Human Geography* 42, no. 6 (2018): 862–80. https://doi.org/10.1177 /0309132517725808.

Plokhy, Serhii. *Chernobyl: The History of a Nuclear Catastrophe.* New York: Basic Books, 2018.

Pohl, Michaela. "From White Grave to Tselinograd to Astana: The Virgin Lands Opening, Khrushchev's Forgotten First Reform." In *The Thaw: Soviet Society and Culture during the 1950s and 1960s,* edited by Denis Kozlov and Eleonory Gilburd, 269–307. Toronto: University of Toronto Press, 2013.

– "The 'Planet of One Hundred Languages': Ethnic Relation and Soviet Identity in the Virgin Lands." In *Peopling the Russian Periphery: Borderland Colonization in Eurasian History,* edited by N. Breyfogle, A. Shrader, and W. Sunderland, 238–61. London: Routledge, 2007.

Polese, Abel. "What Is Informality? (Mapping) 'the Art of Bypassing the State' in Eurasian Spaces – and Beyond." *Eurasian Geography and Economics* 64, no. 3 (2021): 322–64. https://doi.org/10.1080/15387216.2021.1992791.

Polleri, Maxime. "Post-Political Uncertainties: Governing Nuclear Controversies in Post-Fukushima Japan." *Social Science Studies* 50, no. 4 (2020): 567–88. https://doi.org/10.1177/0306312719889405.

Prentice, Rebecca. "Work after Precarity: Anthropologies of Labor and Wageless Life." *Focaal – Journal of Global and Historical Anthropology* 88 (2020): 117–24. https://doi.org/10.3167/fcl.2020.880108.

Prime Minister of the Republic of Kazakhstan. "In Kazakhstan, Over the Past 20 Years, Mortality from Cancer Has Decreased by 33%." Last modified February 28, 2023. https://primeminister.kz/ru/news/v-kazakhstane-za-poslednie-20 -let-smertnost-ot-onkologicheskikh-zabolevaniy-snizilas-na-33-23189.

Purvis-Roberts, K., Werner C., and Frank, I. "Perceived Risks from Radiation and Nuclear Testing Near Semipalatinsk, Kazakhstan: A Comparison Between Physicians, Scientists, and the Public." *Risk Analysis* 27, no. 2 (2007): 291–302. https://doi.org/10.1111/j.1539-6924.2007.00882.x.

Rabinow, Paul. *Essays on the Anthropology of Reason.* Princeton, NJ: Princeton University Press, 1996.

Rechel, Bernd, Erica Richardson, and Martin McKee, eds. *Trends in Health Systems in the Former Soviet Countries.* Copenhagen: World Health Organization on behalf of the European Observatory on Health Systems and Policies, 2014.

Rechel, B., M. Ahmedov, B. Akkazieva, A. Katsaga, G. Khodjamurodov, M. McKee. "Lessons from Two Decades of Health Reform in Central Asia." *Health Policy and Planning* 27, no. 4 (2012): 281–87. https://doi.org/10.1093 /heapol/czr040.

Radiation Effects Research Foundation. "Genetic Effects of Radiation in the Offspring of Atomic-Bomb Survivors." Accessed February 15, 2015. https:// www.rerf.or.jp/en/programs/roadmap_e/health_effects-en/geneefx-en/.

Reeves, Madeleine. *Border Work: Spatial Lives of the State in Rural Central Asia.* Ithaca, NY: Cornell University Press, 2014.

Renfrew, Daniel. *Life Without Lead: Contamination, Crisis, and Hope in Uruguay.* Oakland: University of California Press, 2018.

Resnick, Elana. "The Limits of Resilience: Managing Waste in the Racialized Anthropocene." *American Anthropologist* 123, no. 2 (2021): 222–36. https:// doi.org/10.1111/aman.13542.

Rivkin-Fish, Michelle. *Women's Health in Post-Soviet Russia: The Politics of Intervention.* Bloomington, IN: Indiana University Press, 2005.

Rogers, Douglas. *The Depths of Russia: Oil, Power, and Culture after Socialism.* Ithaca, NY: Cornell University Press, 2015.

Rose, Nickolas. *The Politics of Life Itself: Biomedicine, Power, and Subjectivity in the Twenty-First Century.* Princeton. NJ: Princeton University Press, 2006.

Roudakova, Natalia, and Deborah Ballard-Reisch. "Femininity and the Double Burden: Dialogues on the Socialization of Russian Daughters into Womanhood." *Anthropology of East Europe Review* 17, no. 1 (1999): 21–34. https://scholarworks.iu.edu/journals/index.php/aeer/article/view /536/639.

Rumyantsev, A. "Remarks by the Minister of the Russian Federation for Atomic Energy." In *Security of Radioactive Sources*. Vienna: IAEA, 2003.

Saktaganova, Zauresh. *Sovetskaia Moderniza Ekonomiki Kazakhstana v 1946–70 gg: Kritika Istorichiskogo Opyta* [Soviet Economic Modernization of Kazakhstan in 1946–70] Karaganda, Kazakhstan: Glasir, 2012.

Sarsembaev, Azamat. "Imagined Communities: Kazak Nationalism and Kazakification in the 1990s." *Central Asian Survey* 18, no. 3 (1999): 319–46. https://doi.org/10.1080/02634939995605.

Scheper-Hughes, Nancy. *Death without Weeping: The Violence of Everyday Life in Brazil*. Berkeley: University of California Press, 1992.

– "Mr. Tati's Holiday and João's Safari – Seeing the World through Transplant Tourism." *Body and Society* 17, no. 2–3 (2011): 55–92. https://doi.org/10.1177/1357034x11402858.

– "The Primacy of the Ethical: Propositions for a Militant Anthropology." *Current Anthropology* 36, no. 3 (1995): 409–40. https://doi.org/10.1086/204378.

– *Saints, Scholars, and Schizophrenics: Mental Illness in Rural Ireland*. Berkeley: University of California Press, 1982.

– "A Talent for Life: Reflections on Human Vulnerability and Resilience." *Ethnos* 73, no. 1 (2008): 25–56. https://doi.org/10.1080/00141840801927525.

Schatz, Edward. *Modern Clan Politics: The Power of "Blood" in Kazakhstan and Beyond*. Seattle: University of Washington Press, 2004.

– 'Notes on the 'Dog That Didn't Bark': Eco-Internationalism in Late Soviet Kazakhstan." *Ethnic and Racial Studies Review* 22, no. 2 (1999): 136–61. https://doi.org/10.1080/014198799329620.

Scott, James. *Weapons of the Weak: Everyday Forms of Peasant Resistance*. New Haven, CT: Yale University Press, 1985.

Semenova, Yuliya, Ludmila Pivina, Almira Manatova, Geir Bjorklund, Natalya Glushkova, Tatyana Belikhina, Marzhan Dauletyarova, and Tamara Zhunussova. "Mental Distress in the Rural Kazakhstani Population Exposed and Non-Exposed to Radiation from the Semipalatinsk Nuclear Test Site." *Journal of Environmental Radioactivity* 203 (2019): 39–47. https://doi.org/10.1016/j.jenvrad.2019.02.013.

Semioshkina, N., and Voigt, G. 2006. "An Overview on GSF Activities at the Semipalatinsk Test Site, Kazakhstan." *Journal of Radiation Research* 47, Supplement A, A95–A100. https://doi.org/10.1269/jrr.47.a95.

Shaw, Ian, and Marv Waterstone. *Wageless Life: A Manifesto for a Future beyond Capitalism*. Minneapolis: University of Minnesota Press, 2019.

Shedenova, Nazym, and Aigul Beimisheva. "Social and Economic Status of Urban and Rural Households in Kazakhstan." *Procedia-Social and Behavioral Sciences* 82 (2013): 585–91.

Simpson, Audra. "Consent's Revenge." *Cultural Anthropology* 31, no. 3 (2016): 326–33. https://doi.org/10.14506/ca31.3.02.

– *Mohawk Interruptus: Political Life Across the Borders of Settler States*. Durham, NC: Duke University Press, 2014.

– "On Ethnographic Refusal: Indigeneity, 'Voice' and Colonial Citizenship." *Junctures* 9 (2007): 67–80. https://doi.org/10.34074/junc.20017.

Solzhenitsyn, Aleksander. *The Gulag Archipelago*. New York: Harper & Row, 1973.

Sontag, Susan. *Regarding the Pain of Others*. New York: Farrar, Straus and Giroux, 2003.

Spankulova, Lazat, Marat Karatayev, and Michèle Clarke. "Trends in Socioeconomic Health Inequalities in Kazakhstan: National Household Surveys Analysis." *Communist and Post-Communist Studies* 53, no. 2 (2020): 177–90. https://doi.org/10.1525/cpcs.2020.53.2.177.

Spravochnik, Spravochnik po Istorii Kolkhozov, Sovkhozov i Drugikh Sel'skokhoziastvennykh Predpriiatii Karagandinskoi Oblasti [Handbook, handbook of the history of Kolkhozes, Sovkhozes and other agricultural enterprises of the Karaganda region]. Karaganda, Kazakhstan: Odtel Arkhivov i Dokumentov Karagandinskoi Oblasti, 2012.

Starks, Tricia. *The Body Soviet: Propaganda, Hygiene, and the Revolutionary State*. Madison: University of Wisconsin Press, 2008.

Stawkowski, Magdalena. "Life on an Atomic Collective. The Post-Soviet Retreat of the State in Rural Kazakhstan." *Études Rurales* 200, no. 2 (2018): 196–219.

– "Radiophobia Had to Be Reinvented." *Culture, Theory and Critique* 58, no. 4 (2017): 357–74.

Stephens, Sharon. "The 'Cultural Fallout' of Chernobyl Radiation in Norwegian Sami Regions: Implications for Children." In *Children and the Politics of Culture*, edited by Sharon Stephens, 292–318. Princeton, NJ: Princeton University Press,1995.

Sternsdorff-Cisterna, Nicolas. *Food Safety after Fukushima: Scientific Citizenship and the Politics of Risk*. Honolulu: University of Hawai'i Press, 2019.

Sturgatsky, Arkady, and Boris Strugatsky. *Roadside Picnic*. London: Gollancz, 2007 [1972].

Sultangazin, U.M., E.A. Zakharin, L.F. Spivak, O.P. Arhipkin, N.R. Muratova, A.G. Terehov. "Distantsionnoe Zondirovanie Temperaturnykh Anomalii v Raione Semipalatinskogo Iadernogo Poligona" [Remote sensing of thermal anomalies at the territory of the Semipalatinsk test site]" *Lectures of Ministry of Science of the Academy of Science of the Republic of Kazakhstan* 6, no. 2 (1997): 51–54.

Szymborska, Wisława. *Miracle Fair: Selected Poems of Wisława Szymborska*. Translated by Joanna Trzeciak. New York: W.W. Norton, 2001.

Tabyshalieva, Anara. "Revival of Traditions in Post-Soviet Central Asia." In *Making the Transition Work for Women in Europe and Central Asia*, edited by Marnia Lazreg. World Bank Discussion Paper no. 411, Europe and Central Asia Gender and Development Series. Washington, DC: World Bank, 2000.

Taussig, Michael. *The Devil and Commodity Fetishism in South America*. Chapel Hill: University of North Carolina Press, 1980.

Timonova, Lyubov, Natalia Larinova, Almira Aidarkhanova, Oxana Lyakhova, Medet Aktayev, Zarina Serzhanova, Sergey Lukashenko, Vasiliy Polevik, Alexey Dashuk, Valeriy Monayenko Sergey Subbotin, and Assan Aidarkhanov. "Tritium Distribution in the 'Water-Soil-Air' System in the Semipalatinsk Test Site." *PLoS ONE* 19, no. 4 (2024): e0297017. https://doi.org/10.1371/journal.pone.0297017.

Trouillot, Michel. *Silencing the Past: Power and the Production of History*. Boston, MA: Beacon Press, 1995.

Tsing, Anna. *The Mushroom at the End of the World: On the Possibility of Life in Capitalist Ruins*. Princeton, NJ: Princeton University Press, 2015.

Turaeva, Rano. "Informal Economies in Post-Soviet Space: Post-Soviet Islam and Its Role in Ordering Entrepreneurship in Central Asia." *Central Asian Affairs* 5, no. 1 (2018): 57–75. https://doi.org/10.1163/22142290-00501004.

UNHRC (United Nations Human Rights Council). *Report of the Special Rapporteur on the Implications for Human Rights of the Environmentally Sound Management and Disposal of Hazardous Substances and Wastes: Mission to Kazakhstan. United Nations General Assembly*. Geneva: United Nations, 2015.

United Nations. *United Nations in Kazakhstan Annual Report 2021*. Geneva: United Nations, 2021.

USNRC (United States Nuclear Regulatory Commission). 'Backgrounder on Biological Effects of Radiation.' *United States Nuclear Regulatory Commission*, 2015. https://www.nrc.gov/reading-rm/doc-collections/fact-sheets/bio-effects-radiation.html.

Vakulchuk, Roman, and Kristian Gjerde, with Tatiana Belkhina and Kazbek Apsalikov. *Semipalatinsk Nuclear Testing: The Humanitarian Consequences*. Report 1. Oslo: Norwegian Institute of International Affairs, 2014.

Veber, Elena. "Zhitelia Karagandy Neskol'ko Raz Pereprodavali v Rabstvo" [A resident of Karaganda was resold into slavery several times]. *Radio Azattyk*, March 29, 2012, https://rus.azattyq.org/a/rabstvo_vladimir_temirtau_tarabukina_/24530747.html.

Velikanov, Aleksander E. "About the Nature of Regional Thermal Anomaly in Semipalatinsk Test Site Region." *Mathematics and Computers in Simulation* 67, no. 4–5 (2004): 459–65. https://doi.org/10.1016/j.matcom.2004.06.024.

Verdery, Katherine. *What Was Socialism, and What Comes Next?* Princeton, NJ: Princeton University Press, 1996.

Viola, Lynne. *Peasant Rebels Under Stalin: Collectivization and the Culture of Peasant Resistance*. Oxford: Oxford University Press, 1996.

– *The Unknown Gulag: The Lost World of Stalin's Special Settlements*. New York: Oxford University Press, 2007.

Volodine, Antoine. *Radiant Terminus*. Rochester, NY: Open Letter, 2017.

Voyles, Traci. *Wastelanding: Legacies of Uranium Mining in Navajo Country.* Minneapolis: University of Minnesota Press, 2015.

Vries de, Pieter, and Han Seur. *Mururoa and Us: Polynesians' Experiences during Thirty Years of Nuclear Testing in the French Pacific.* Lyon: Centre de Documentation et de Recherchere sur la Paix et les Conflics, 1997.

Walker, Charles. "Space, Kinship Networks and Youth Transition in Provincial Russia: Negotiating Urban-Rural and Inter-Regional Migration." *Europe-Asia Studies* 62, no. 4 (2020): 647–69. https://doi.org/10.1080/09668131003736995.

Walker, J. Samuel. "The Atomic Energy Commission and the Politics of Radiation Protection, 1967–1971." *Isis* 85, no. 1 (1994): 57–78. https://doi.org/10.1086/356727.

Weinbert, H., A. Korol, V. Kirzhner, A. Avivi, T. Fahima, E. Nevo, S. Shapiro, G. Rennert, O. Piatek, E. Stepanova, and E. Skvarskaja. "Very High Mutation Rate in Offspring of Chernobyl Accident Liquidators." *Proceedings of the Royal Society B.* 268, no. 1471 (2001): 1471–2954. https://doi.org/10.1098/rspb.2001.1650.

Werner, Cynthia. "Bride Abduction in Post-Soviet Central Asia: Marking a Shift Towards Patriarchy through Local Discourses of Shame and Tradition." *The Journal of the Royal Anthropological Institute* 15, no. 2 (2009): 314–31. https://doi.org/10.1111/j.1467-9655.2009.01555.x.

– "Women, Marriage, and the Nation-State: The Rise of Nonconsensual Bride Kidnapping in Post-Soviet Kazakhstan." In *The Transformation of Central Asia: States and Societies from Soviet Rule to Independence,* edited by Pauline Jones-Luong, 59–90. Ithaca, NY: Cornell University Press, 2004.

Werner, Cynthia, Christopher Edling, Charles Becker, Elena Kim, Russell Kleinbach, Fatima Esengeldievna Sartbay, and Woden Teachout. "Bride Kidnapping in Post-Soviet Eurasia: A Roundtable Discussion." *Central Asian Survey* 37, no. 4 (2018): 582–601. https://doi.org/10.1080/02634937.2018.1511519.

Werner, Cynthia, and Holly Barcus. "The Unequal Burdens of Repatriation: A Gendered view of the Transnational Migration of Mongolia's Kazakh Population." *American Anthropologist* 117, no. 2 (2015): 257–71. https://doi.org/10.1111/aman.12230

Werner, Cynthia, and Kathleen Purvis-Roberts. "After the Cold War: International Politics, Domestic Policy and the Nuclear Legacy in Kazakhstan." *Central Asian Survey* 25, no. 4 (2006): 461–80. https://doi.org/10.1080/02634930701210542.

– "Cold War Memories and Post–Cold War Realities: The Politics of Memory and Identity in the Everyday Life of Kazakhstan's Radiation Victims." In *The Anthropology of the State in Central Asia,* edited by Madeleine Reeves, Johan Rasanayagam, and Judith Beyer, 285–309. Bloomington, IN: Indiana University Press, 2014.

– "Unraveling the Secrets of the Past: Contested Versions of Nuclear Testing in the Soviet Republic of Kazakhstan." In *Half-Lives and Half-Truths: Confronting the Radioactive Legacies of the Cold War,* edited by Barbara Rose Johnston, 277–98. Santa Fe, NM: School for Advanced Research Press, 2007.

Wertelecki, Wladimir. "Malformations in A Chernobyl-Impacted Region." *Pediatrics* 125, no. 4 (2010): e836–e843. https://doi.org/10.1542/peds.2009-2219.

Wheeler, William. *Environment and Post-Soviet Transformation in Kazakhstan's Aral Sea Region: Sea Changes.* London: UCL Press, 2021.

WHO (World Health Organization). *Health Systems in Action: Kazakhstan.* Geneva: WHO, 2022. https://eurohealthobservatory.who.int/publications/i/health-systems-in-action-kazakhstan-2022.

Williams, Raymond. *The Country and the City.* London: Chatto and Windus, 1973.

World Bank. *Doing Business 2020: Comparing Business Regulation in 190 Economies.* Washington, DC: International Bank for Reconstruction and Development/The World Bank, 2020. https://openknowledge.worldbank.org/server/api/core/bitstreams/75ea67f9-4bcb-5766-ada6-6963a992d64c/content.

– *Macro Poverty Outlook: Kazakhstan.* Washington, DC: World Bank, 2022. https://thedocs.worldbank.org/en/doc/d5f32ef28464d01f195827b7e020a3e8-0500022021/related/mpo-kaz.pdf.

– *World Bank Group-Kazakhstan Partnership Program Snapshot.* Astana, Kazakhstan: World Bank, 2015. https://www.worldbank.org/content/dam/Worldbank/document/Kazakhstan-Snapshot.pdf.

World Nuclear Association. *Uranium and Nuclear Power in Kazakhstan.* London: World Nuclear Association, 2023. https://world-nuclear.org/information-library/country-profiles/countries-g-n/kazakhstan.aspx.

Wynne, Brian. *Rationality and Ritual: Participation and Exclusion in Nuclear-Decision Making.* 2nd ed. London: Earthscan, 2011.

Yan, Wudan. "The Nuclear Sins of the Soviet Union Live on in Kazakhstan." *Nature,* April 3, 2019. https://www.nature.com/articles/d41586-019-01034-8.

Yeager, Meredith, Mitchell J. Machiela, Prachi Kothiyal, Michael Dean, Clara Bodelon, Shalabh Suman, Mingyi Wang, et al. "Lack of Transgenerational Effects of Ionizing Radiation Exposure from Chernobyl Accident." *Science* 375, no. 6543 (2021): 725–29. https://doi.org/10.1126/science.abg2365.

Yessenova, Saulesh. *The Politics and Poetics of the Nation: Urban Narratives of Kazakh Identity.* Saarbrücken, Germany: LAP Lambert Academic Publishing, 2010.

– "Routes and Roots of Kazakh Identity, Germany: Urban Migration in Postsocialist Kazakhstan." *Russian Review* 64, no. 4 (2005): 661–79. https://doi.org/10.1111/j.1467-9434.2005.00380.x.

"The Tengiz Oil Enclave: Labor, Business, and the State." *Polar* 35, no. 1 (2012): 94–114. https://doi.org/10.1111/j.1555-2934.2012.01181.x.

Yevelson, Ilya I., Anna Abdelgani, Julie Cwikel, and Igor S. Yevelson. "Bridging the Gap in Mental Health Approaches between East and West: The Psychosocial Consequences of Radiation Exposure." *Environmental Health Perspectives* 105, Suppl. 6 (1997): 1551–56. https://doi.org/10.2307/3433669.

Zakarin, Edige, Larissa Balakay, Bibigul Mirkarimova, Natalia Tuseeva, Konstantin Pak, Alexander Baklanovm, Alexander Mahura, Jens H. Sorensen. *Geoinformation Modeling of Radionuclide Transfer from the Territory of the Semipalatinsk Test Site: FP6 EC CA – Enviro-RISKS: Man-Induced Environmental Risks: Monitoring, Management and Radiation of Man-made Changes in Siberia.* Copenhagen: Danish Meteorological Institute, 2008.

Zalasiewicz, Jan, Mark Williams, Will Steffen, Paul Crutzen. "The New World of the Anthropocene." *Environmental Science and Technology* 44, no. 7 (2010): 2228–31. https://doi.org/10.1021/es903118j.

Zimovina, E.P. "Dinamika Chislennosti i Sostava Naseleniia Kazakhstana vo Vtoroi Polovine KhKh Veka." *Demoskop Weekly*, no. 103–104 (2003). http://www.demoscope.ru/weekly/2003/0103/analit03.php.

Zhumadilov, Zhaxybay, Boris I. Gusev, Jun Takada, Masaharu Hoshi, Akiro Kimura, Norihiko Hayakawa, and Nobuo Takeichi. "Thyroid Abnormality Trend Over Time in Northeastern Regions of Kazakstan, Adjacent to the Semipalatinsk Nuclear Test Site: A Case Review of Pathological Findings for 7271 Patients." *Journal of Radiation Research* 41, no. 1 (2000): 35–44. https://doi.org/10.1269/jrr.41.35.

Index

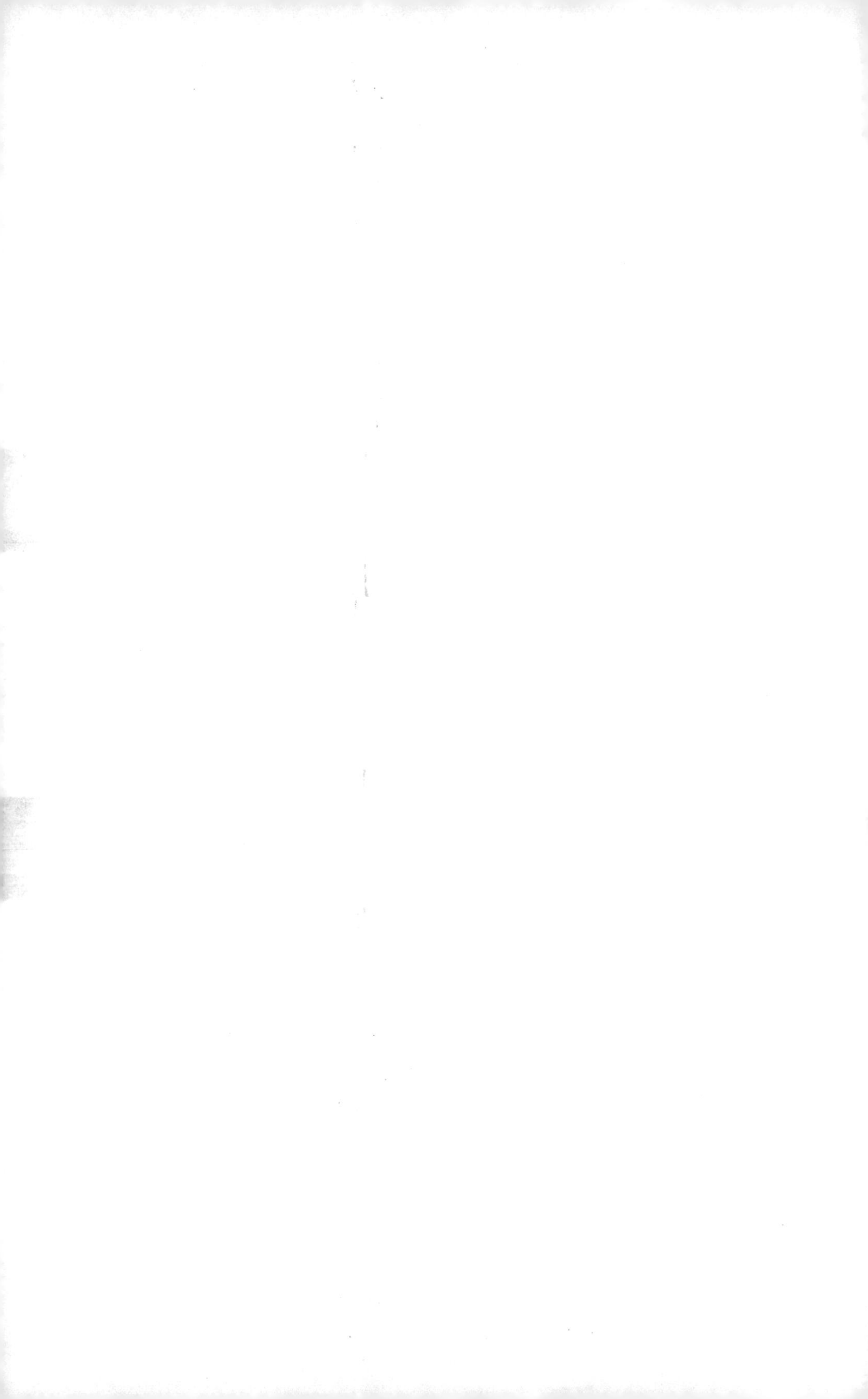